Sirtfoo

A Nutritional Guide For Beginners With Healthy Recipes To Activate Your Skinny Gene And Metabolism With The Help Of Sirt Foods And Burn Fat.

Dr I. Pot

Table of Contents

INTRODUCTION

Regardless of whether you're attempting to get in shape or getting increasingly careful about energizing your body, it's essential to comprehend Sirtfoods. Sirtfoods are a gathering of nourishments wealthy in supplements that help manage your digestion, consume fat, and increment muscle. Aidan Goggins and Glen Matten, creators of THE SIRTFOOD DIET, share what you have to think about Sirtfoods.

When we cut back on calories, it makes a lack of vitality that enacts what is known as the "thin quality." This triggers a heap of positive changes. It places the body into a sort of endurance mode where it quits putting away fat and ordinary development forms are required to be postponed momentarily. Rather, the body directs its concentration toward consuming its stores of fat and turning on amazing housekeeping qualities that fix and restore our phones, successfully giving them a spring cleaning. The end result is weight loss and improved protection from ailment.

Be that as it may, the same number of dieters knows, cutting calories includes some significant downfalls. Temporarily, the decrease in vitality consumption incites hunger, crabbiness, weakness, and muscle loss. Longer-term calorie limitation makes our digestion stagnate. This is the defeat of all calorie-prohibitive diets and makes ready for the weight to return heaping on. It is thus that 99 percent of dieters are destined to bomb over the long haul.

The entirety of this drove us to pose a major inquiry: is it by one way or another conceivable to actuate our thin quality with all the extraordinary advantages that brings without expecting to adhere to exceptional calorie limitation with every one of those downsides?

Enter Sirtfoods, a newfound gathering of marvel nourishments. Sirtfoods are especially wealthy in uncommon supplements that, when we expend them, can initiate similar thin qualities in our bodies that calorie limitation does. These qualities are known as sirtuins. They previously became known in a milestone study in 2003 when scientists found that resveratrol, a compound found in red grape skin and red wine, significantly expanded the life range of yeast.[2] Incredibly, resveratrol had a similar impact on life span as calorie limitation, yet this was accomplished without lessening vitality admission. From that point forward investigations have indicated that resveratrol can expand

life in worms, flies, fish, and even honeybees.3 And from mice to people, beginning time examines show resveratrol secures against the unfriendly impacts of unhealthy, high-fat, and high-sugar diets; advances sound maturing by deferring age-related sicknesses; and increments fitness.4 basically it has been appeared to impersonate the impacts of calorie limitation and exercise.

With its rich resveratrol content, red wine was hailed as the first Sirtfood, clarifying the medical advantages connected to its utilization, and even why individuals who drink red wine increase less weight. However, this is just the start of the Sirtfood story.

With the revelation of resveratrol, the universe of wellbeing research was on the cusp of something significant, and the pharmaceutical business burned through no time committing. Scientists started screening a huge number of different synthetic substances for their capacity to initiate our sirtuin qualities. This uncovered various characteristic plant mixes, not only resveratrol, with significant sirtuin-actuating properties. It was additionally found that a given nourishment could contain an entire range of these plant mixes, which could work in show to both guide retention and amplify that nourishment's sirtuin-enacting impact. This had been one of the huge riddles around resveratrol. The researchers trying different things with resveratrol often expected to use far higher dosages than we know give an advantage when expended as a major aspect of red wine. In any case, just as resveratrol, red wine contains a variety of other regular plant mixes, including high measures of piceatannol just as quercetin, myricetin, and epicatechin, every one of which was appeared to autonomously initiate our sirtuin qualities and, progressively significant, to work in coordination.

The issue for the pharmaceutical business is that they can't advertise a gathering of supplements or nourishments as the following huge blockbuster sedate. So all things being equal they contributed a huge number of dollars to create and direct preliminaries of manufactured mixes with expectations of revealing a Shangri-la pill. At this moment various investigations of sirtuin-enacting drugs are in progress for a huge number of interminable maladies, just as the first-since forever FDA-endorsed preliminary to examine whether a prescription can slow maturing.

As tempting as that may appear, if history has shown us anything, it's that we ought not to hold out a lot of trust in this pharmaceutical ambrosia. Consistently the pharmaceutical and wellbeing enterprises have attempted to copy the advantages of nourishments and diets through segregated medications and supplements. What's more, on numerous occasions it's missed the mark. Why sit tight ten or more years for the permitting of these supposed marvel drugs, and the unavoidable reactions they bring, when right now we have all the staggering advantages accessible readily available through the nourishment we eat?

So while the pharmaceutical business perseveringly seeks after a drug like enchantment slug, we need to retrain our emphasis on diet.

WHAT ARE SIRTFOOD?

While the world has been hanging tight for Adele to drop new music, it's been getting only somewhat fixated on her weight. There's no uncertainty that she looks extraordinary (um, hasn't she generally?) and it's reputed to be down to the Sirtfood Diet.

Lexi Larson, a 19-year-old from Hingham, Massachusetts, revealed to People that she met Adele on an extended get-away in Anguilla and that the music whiz disclosed to her she had "lost something like 100 pounds," portraying it as an "insane constructive encounter."

Adele hasn't affirmed that her weight loss is down to the Sirtfood Diet (or some other diet); however she is highlighted on the authority Sirtfood Diet site with the words, "Adele's top-mystery fat-softening diet."

So what's the serious deal about the Sirtfood Diet?

The eating plan depends on polyphenols, characteristic mixes found in plant nourishments that help to shield the cells in the body from aggravation or demise through sickness. According to wellbeing advisors Aidan Goggins and Glen Matten, who formulated the Sirtfood

Diet, a little gathering of polyphenols can imitate the impacts of fasting and exercise by initiating the body's sirtuin (otherwise known as "thin") qualities.

"In view of expending a specific rundown of solid, polyphenol-rich nourishments, the Sirtfood Diet guarantees weight and fat decrease without muscle loss," says New York-based dietitian-nutritionist Tanya Freirich, RD, at Sweet Nova.

What's the arrangement?

There are two stages to the Sirtfood diet; the primary goes on for multi week and the second for about fourteen days. During the initial three days of the arrangement, you're confined to 1,000 calories from one feast of sirtfoods and three green juices. For the remainder of the primary week, you can devour two green juices and two sirtfood dinners for every day. During stage two, the day by day feast plan comprises of three sirtfood dinners and one green juice.

Adjusted sirtfood-rich dinners incorporate Asian Shrimp Stir-Fry with Buckwheat Noodles and Strawberry Buckwheat Tabbouleh.

Past the underlying three-week "kick off" period, Goggins and Matten prescribe proceeding to incorporate sirtfoods in your dinners to keep getting results.

What does it guarantee?

"If you don't veer off from the arrangement, the Sirtfood Diet guarantees a seven-pound weight loss in the primary week (without losing bulk)," says Freirich. "It additionally claims to have hostile to maturing impacts, to help improve memory and glucose control and lessen the danger of ceaseless ailment."

In any case, does it convey?

The examination on the job of sirtuin is really meager— for the most part research center investigations including yeast, lab creatures, and human undeveloped cells. One examination, distributed in 2013 in the diary Oxidative Medicine and Cellular Longevity, proposes polyphenol utilization has a similar advantageous impact on human digestion as calorie limitation. However, until this dietary methodology is really tried in human clinical preliminaries, it's difficult to state with any assurance how individuals may toll.

What would you be able to eat?

While some sirtfoods are standard in any grocery store or wellbeing nourishment store (and may as of now be in your kitchen), others may not be so natural to discover.

"Sirtfoods incorporate kale, dull chocolate, red wine, cocoa powder, turmeric, onions, parsley, garlic, pecans, and strawberries," Freirich says. "A large portion of the fixings are anything but difficult to discover and are notable as solid decisions. In any case, extra fixings might be more enthusiastically to source, similar to lovage, buckwheat, and matcha green tea powder."

What wouldn't you be able to eat?

Formally, no nourishments are "prohibited" on the Sirtfood Diet, yet the calorie limitation is not kidding—especially during the underlying three days, when you're constrained to 1,000 calories.

To place that in context, 1,000 calories is the prescribed admission for an inactive 2-to 3-year-old, according to the USDA Dietary Guidelines for 2015-2020,

Are there any disadvantages?

The hardest piece of the Sirtfood Diet is calorie limitation and the dependence on green juice, and this could be perilous for specific gatherings of individuals, Freirich says. She wouldn't prescribe this diet for individuals on certain drugs, similar to Coumadin, or with wellbeing conditions like diabetes. She'd likewise give it a miss if you're preparing broadly or are pregnant or breastfeeding.

"By and large, I don't suggest any diets that depend on excessively prohibitive outside principles," Freirich includes. "Be that as it may, a significant number of the suggested 'sirtfoods' are wellbeing advancing, and I'd prescribe individuals consolidate these in their dinners. As usual, I emphatically urge individuals to tune in to their body's craving and satiety signals for direction on when and how much nourishment to eat."

SHED SEVEN POUNDS IN SEVEN DAYS WITH THE SOLID ROUTE ON THE SIRTFOOD DIET RECIPE

According to an ongoing review, the normal lady increases 5lb in pre-winter, while December is the fattest month of the year.

But if every one of those pumpkin flavor lattes in the course of the most recent couple of months mean you're breaking a rib attempting to press into your LBD in time for the workplace party, the current year's most discussed diet guarantees that you can shed 7lb in only seven days, keep the weight off and still have chocolate.

It might sound unrealistic, however superstars, for example, Adele, Lorraine Pascale and Jodie Kidd depend on the Sirtfood Diet.

"A sirtfood is high in sirtuin activators," clarifies nutritionist Aidan Goggins, co-writer of the top of the line book The Sirtfood Diet.

"Sirtuins are a kind of protein that shields cells from kicking the bucket or getting aggravated. They can likewise launch your digestion, control your hunger, help muscle tone and consume fat."

So how can it work?

"For the initial three days, you confine calorie admission to 1,000 calories every day, which incorporates drinking three sirtfood green juices in addition to eating

A sirtfood-rich feast and nibbling on cell reinforcement stuffed 'sirtfood chomps'," says Aidan.

"Throughout the previous four days, you up the calorie admission to 1,500 calories per day by expending two sirtfood-rich dinners and two green juices, removing the chomps."

What's to come?

You can do this arrangement for as long as about fourteen days, after which it's tied in with modifying it to suit your lifestyle.

"There are no set guidelines – simply attempt to incorporate however many sirtfoods as could be allowed in your diet, which should cause you to feel more beneficial, increasingly vivacious and improve your skin, just as making you more slender," says Aidan.

"Customers who have continued with the diet have seen proceeded and supported weight loss of over 2st."

Your seven-day plan

This super-sound green juice and these yummy choc balls are Sirtfood Diet staples.

All plans serve one (except if in any case expressed).

Sirtfood Green Juice

*75g kale

*30g rocket

*5g level leaf parsley

*5g lovage leaves (discretionary)

*150g celery, including leaves

*1/2 medium green apple

*Juice 1/2 lemon

*1/2tsp matcha green tea

1 Juice the kale, rocket, parsley and lovage, if utilizing, then include the celery and apple and mix once more. Press in the lemon.

2 Pour a modest quantity of the juice into a glass, then include the matcha and mix until broke up. Include the rest of the juice and serve right away.

NOTE only use matcha in the initial two beverages of the day, as it contains a similar caffeine content as a typical cup of tea. If you're not accustomed to it, it might keep you conscious if alcoholic later in the day.

Sirtfood Bites (makes 15-20 chomps)

*120g pecans

*30g dull chocolate (85% cocoa solids), broken into pieces, or cocoa nibs

*250g Medjool dates, pitted

*1tbsp cocoa powder

*1tbsp ground turmeric

*1tbsp additional virgin olive oil

*Scraped seeds of 1 vanilla unit or 1tsp vanilla concentrate

1 Place the pecans and chocolate into a nourishment processor and mix until you have a fine powder. Include the various fixings and mix until the blend shapes an

enormous ball. Add 2tbsp water to help tie it, if required.

2 Using your hands, make scaled down balls from the blend and refrigerate in an impermeable holder for at any rate 1 hour before serving. The balls will keep for as long as seven days in the ice chest.

Day 1

3 x sirtfood green juices

2 x sirtfood chomps (you can substitute these for 15-20g of dull chocolate if you wish)

1 x sirtfood supper

Asian lord prawn pan sear

*150g crude ruler prawns, shelled

*2tsp tamari or soy sauce

*2tsp additional virgin olive oil

*1 clove garlic, finely hacked

*1 10,000 foot stew, finely slashed

*1tsp new ginger, finely hacked

*20g red onion, cut

*40g celery, cut and cut

*75g green beans, hacked

*50g kale, generally hacked

*100ml chicken stock

*75g soba (buckwheat noodles)

*5g lovage or celery leaves

1 In a skillet over a high warmth, cook the prawns in 1tsp tamari or soy sauce and 1tsp oil for 2-3 minutes. Move to a plate.

2 Add the rest of the oil to the dish and fry the garlic, stew, ginger, red onion, celery, beans and kale over a medium-high warmth for 2-3 minutes. Add the stock and bring to the bubble, then stew until the vegetables are cooked yet at the same time crunchy.

3 Cook the noodles in bubbling water according to pack directions. Channel and include the lovage or celery leaves, noodles and prawns to the container. Take back to the bubble, then expel from the warmth and serve.

Day 2

*3 x sirtfood green juices

*2 x sirtfood nibbles

*1 x sirtfood feast

Turkey escalope

*150g cauliflower, generally slashed

*1 clove garlic, finely slashed

*40g red onion, finely slashed

*1 superior stew, finely hacked

*1tsp crisp ginger, finely hacked

*2tbsp additional virgin olive oil

*2tsp ground turmeric

*30g sun-dried tomatoes, finely hacked

*10g parsley

*150g turkey escalope

*1tsp dried sage

*Juice 1/2 lemon

*1tbsp tricks

1 Place the cauliflower in a nourishment processor and heartbeat in 2-second blasts to finely cleave it until it

looks like couscous. Put in a safe spot. Fry the garlic, red onion, bean stew and ginger in 1tsp of the oil until delicate however not hued. Include the turmeric and cauliflower and cook for 1 moment. Expel from the warmth and include the sun-dried tomatoes and a large portion of the parsley.

2 Coat the turkey escalope in the rest of the oil and sage then fry for 5-6 minutes, turning normally. When cooked, include the lemon juice, remaining parsley, tricks and 1tbsp water to the container to make a sauce, then serve.

Day 3

3 x sirtfood green juices

2 x sirtfood chomps

1 x sirtfood dinner

Fragrant chicken

For the salsa

*1 huge tomato

*1 10,000 foot bean stew, finely cleaved

*1tbsp tricks, finely cleaved

*5g parsley, finely hacked

*Juice 1/2 lemon

For the chicken

*120g skinless, boneless chicken bosom

*2tsp ground turmeric

*Juice 1/2 lemon

*1tbsp additional virgin olive oil

*50g kale, hacked

*20g red onion, cut

*1tsp new ginger, finely cleaved

*50g buckwheat

1 Heat the stove to 220ºC/200ºC fan/gas mark 7.

2 To make the salsa, finely slash the tomato, ensuring you keep however much of the fluid as could reasonably be expected. Blend in with the bean stew, tricks, parsley and lemon juice.

3 Marinate the chicken bosom in 1tsp of the turmeric, lemon juice and a large portion of the oil for 5-10 minutes.

4 Heat an ovenproof griddle, include the marinated chicken and cook for a moment on each side until brilliant, then exchange to the broiler for 8-10 minutes or until cooked through. Expel, spread with foil and leave to rest for 5 minutes.

5 Cook the kale in a steamer for 5 minutes. Fry the onion and ginger in the remainder of the oil until delicate yet not shaded, then include the cooked kale and fry for one more moment.

6 Cook the buckwheat according to pack directions with the rest of the turmeric, and serve.

Day 4

2 x sirtfood green juices

2 x sirtfood dinners

Sirt Muesli

*20g buckwheat chips

*10g buckwheat puffs

*15g coconut chips or dried up coconut

*40g Medjool dates, hollowed and hacked

*15g pecans, hacked

*10g cocoa nibs

*100g strawberries, hulled and hacked

*100g plain Greek yogurt (or veggie lover elective, for example, soya or coconut yogurt)

1 Mix the entirety of the fixings together and serve (forgetting about the strawberries and yogurt if not serving straight away).

Sautéed salmon serving of mixed greens

For the dressing

*10g parsley

*Juice 1/2 lemon

*1tbsp tricks

*1tbsp additional virgin olive oil

For the serving of mixed greens

*1/2 avocado, stripped, stoned and diced

*100g cherry tomatoes, divided

*20g red onion, meagerly cut

*50g rocket

*5g celery leaves

*150g skinless salmon filet

*2tsp darker sugar

*70g chicory (head), divided lengthways

1 Heat the broiler to 220ºC/200ºC fan/gas mark 7.

2 To make the dressing, whizz the parsley, lemon juice, tricks and 2tsp oil in a blender until smooth.

3 For the plate of mixed greens, blend the avocado, tomato, red onion, rocket and celery leaves together.

4 Rub the salmon with a little oil and singe it in an ovenproof skillet for a moment. Move to a heating plate and cook in the broiler for 5 minutes.

5 Mix the darker sugar with 1tsp oil and brush it over the cut sides of the chicory. Spot chop sides down in a hot skillet and cook for 2-3 minutes, turning normally. Dress the plate of mixed greens and serve together.

Day 5

2 x sirtfood green juices

2 x sirtfood dinners

Strawberry tabbouleh

*50g buckwheat

*1tbsp ground turmeric

*80g avocado

*65g tomato

*20g red onion

*25g Medjool dates, pitted

*1tbsp tricks

*30g parsley

*100g strawberries, hulled

*1tbsp additional virgin olive oil

*Juice 1/2 lemon

*30g rocket

1 Cook the buckwheat with the turmeric according to pack guidelines. Channel and cool.

2 Finely cleave the avocado, tomato, red onion, dates, tricks and parsley and blend in with the cooled buckwheat.

3 Slice the strawberries and delicately blend into the plate of mixed greens with the oil and lemon juice. Serve on the rocket.

Miso-marinated prepared cod

*20g miso

*1tbsp mirin

*1tbsp additional virgin olive oil

*200g skinless cod filet

*20g red onion, cut

*40g celery, cut

*1 clove garlic, finely hacked

*1 10,000 foot bean stew, finely cleaved

*1tsp new ginger, finely slashed

*60g green beans

*50g kale, generally hacked

*30g buckwheat

*1tsp ground turmeric

*1tsp sesame seeds

*5g parsley, generally hacked

*1tbsp tamari or soy sauce

1 Heat the stove to 220ºC/200ºC fan/gas mark 7.

2 Mix the miso, mirin and 1tsp oil, rub into the cod and marinate for 30 minutes. Move on to a heating plate and cook for 10 minutes.

3 Meanwhile, heat an enormous skillet with the rest of the oil. Include the onion and sautéed food for a couple of moments, then include the celery, garlic, stew, ginger, green beans and kale. Fry until the kale is delicate and cooked through, adding a little water to soften the kale if required.

4 Cook the buckwheat according to pack directions with the turmeric. Include the sesame seeds, parsley and tamari or soy sauce

To the pan fried food and present with the greens and fish.

Day 6

2 x sirtfood green juices

2 x sirtfood dinners

Sirt super plate of mixed greens

*50g rocket

*50g chicory leaves

*100g smoked salmon cuts

*80g avocado, stripped, stoned and cut

*40g celery, cut

*20g red onion, cut

*15g pecans, hacked

*1tbsp tricks

*1 huge Medjool date, hollowed and slashed

*1tbsp additional virgin olive oil

*Juice 1/2 lemon

*10g parsley, cleaved

*10g lovage or celery leaves, cleaved

1 Mix every one of the fixings together and serve.

Char grilled meat

*100g potatoes, stripped and diced into 2cm 3D shapes

*1tbsp additional virgin olive oil

*5g parsley, finely cleaved

*50g red onion, cut into rings

*50g kale, cleaved

*1 clove garlic, finely cleaved

*120-150g 3.5cm-thick meat filet

Steak or 2cm-thick sirloin steak

*40ml red wine

*150ml meat stock

*1tsp tomato purée

*1tsp corn flour, broke down in 1tbsp water

1 Heat the stove to 220ºC/200ºC fan/gas mark 7.

2 Place the potatoes in a pan of bubbling water, bring to the bubble and cook for 4-5 minutes, then channel. Spot in a simmering tin with 1tsp oil and cook for 35-45 minutes, turning at regular intervals. Expel from the stove, sprinkle with the cleaved parsley and blend well.

3 Fry the onion in 1tsp oil over a medium warmth until delicate and caramelized. Keep warm.

4 Steam the kale for 2-3 minutes, then channel. Fry the garlic delicately in 1/2tsp oil for 1 moment until delicate. Include the kale and fry for a further 1-2 minutes, until delicate. Keep warm.

5 Heat an ovenproof griddle until smoking. Coat the meat in 1/2tsp oil and fry according to how you like your meat done. Expel from the dish and put aside to rest. Add the wine to the hot skillet to raise any meat buildup. Air pocket to decrease the wine considerably until it's syrupy with a concentrated flavor.

6 Add the stock and tomato purée to the steak container and bring to the bubble, then add the corn flour glue to thicken the sauce a little at once until you have the ideal consistency. Mix in any juice from the refreshed steak and present with the potatoes, kale, onion rings and red wine sauce.

Day 7

2 x sirtfood green juices

2 x sirtfood dinners

Sirtfood omelet

*50g streaky bacon

*3 medium eggs

*35g red chicory, daintily cut

*5g parsley, finely cleaved

*1tsp additional virgin olive oil

1 Heat a non-stick skillet. Cut the bacon into slight strips and cook over a high warmth until fresh. You don't have to include any oil – there ought to be sufficient fat in the bacon to cook it. Expel from the dish and spot on kitchen paper to deplete any abundance fat. Wipe the container clean.

2 Whisk the eggs and blend in with the chicory and parsley. Mix the cooked bacon through the eggs.

3 Heat the oil in a non-stick griddle before including the egg blend. Cook until the omelet solidifies. Facilitate the spatula around the edges and overlay the omelet down the middle or move up and serve.

Prepared chicken bosom

For the pesto

*15g parsley

*15g pecans

*15g Parmesan

*1tbsp additional virgin olive oil

*Juice 1/2 lemon

For the chicken

*150g skinless chicken bosom

*20g red onions, finely cut

*1tsp red wine vinegar

*35g rocket

*100g cherry tomatoes, split

*1tsp balsamic vinegar

1 Heat the stove to 220ºC/200ºC fan/gas mark 7.

2 To make the pesto, mix the parsley, pecans, Parmesan, olive oil, a large portion of the lemon juice and 1tbsp water in a nourishment processor until you have

A smooth glue. Step by step include more water until you have your favored consistency.

3 Marinate the chicken bosom in 1tbsp of the pesto and the rest of the lemon squeeze in the cooler for 30 minutes, or more if conceivable.

4 In an ovenproof griddle over a medium-high warmth, fry the chicken in its marinade for 1 moment on either side, then exchange the skillet to the stove and cook for 8 minutes, or until cooked through.

5 Marinate the onions in the red wine vinegar for 5-10 minutes, then channel off the fluid.

6 When the chicken is cooked, expel it from the stove, spoon over 1tbsp pesto and let the warmth from the chicken dissolve the pesto. Spread with foil and leave to rest for 5 minutes before serving.

7 Combine the rocket, tomatoes and onion and shower over the balsamic. Present with the chicken, spooning throughout the remainder of the pesto.

Need to continue onward? Throughout the following 14 days, have 1 x green juice and 3 x sirtfood-rich dinners daily.

Sirtfood Diet For Weight Loss: Lose 3 Kgs In A Week With This Diet Which Allows Red Wine And Chocolate! Sirtfood diet for weight loss: Turmeric, onion, dim chocolate, red wine, dates, pecans and buckwheat are a portion of the nourishments you can eat right now. Peruse here to know how it can assist you with weight loss

It depends on eating a gathering of nourishments that contain something the creators portray as 'sirtuin activators'. Sirtuins are a class of protein, seven of which (SIRT1 to SIRT7) have been identified in people. They seem to have a wide scope of jobs in our body, including potential enemy of maturing and metabolic impacts.

As researchers see progressively about sirtuins, they're getting inspired by the job they may play in assisting with turning on those weight-loss pathways that are generally activated by an absence of nourishment and by taking activity. The hypothesis goes that if you can initiate a portion of the seven sirtuins, you could assist with consuming fat and treat corpulence with less exertion than it takes to follow some different diets or go through hours on the treadmill.

What does it include?

The Sirtfood Diet has two phases. On every one of the initial three days you drink three 'sirt juices' and have one feast (aggregate of 1,000 calories per day). On the accompanying four days you're permitted two sirt juices and two suppers every day (aggregate of 1,500 calories day by day). You then advancement to the simpler stage two, with one juice and three 'adjusted' suppers, in reasonable segment measures, a day.

What would you be able to eat on the diet?

There's a rundown of nourishments containing synthetic exacerbates that the creators state switch on sirtuin and wrench up fat consuming while at the same time bringing down hunger (the last presumably through assisting with accomplishing better glucose control).

Nourishments include: strawberries, pecans, parsley, kale, rocket, espresso, green tea, turmeric, soy, escapades, 10,000 foot chillies, red onion, extra-virgin olive oil, celery, medjool dates, buckwheat, red wine – and, the most well known sirtfood on the square, cocoa (deciphered, obviously, into dull chocolate). Sirt juices are produced using kale, celery, apple, lemon, matcha green tea, rocket and parsley. Run of the mill fundamental dinners incorporate Asian lord prawn pan sear with buckwheat noodles, and kale and red onion dahl with buckwheat.

Is it powerful for weight loss?

You ought to get in shape basically on the grounds that you're eating less calories, particularly in stage one. Without a doubt, you may consume fat quicker with this diet than with 'any old calorie-limited' plan and you may feel more full. With respect to the creators' case this diet is 'clinically demonstrated to lose 7lb in seven days'...

All things considered, it's significant that so far the diet has just been tried on 40 solid, exceptionally energetic human guinea pigs in an upmarket rec center in London's Knightsbridge. The analyzers lost a normal of 7lb in seven days, while indicating increments in bulk and vitality. In any case, then given the calorie limitations of that first week, weight loss may basically be because of the outrageous decrease in calories.

The decision

Further examinations are expected to identify the long haul sway on waistlines – and general wellbeing – and to see whether sirt dieters keep the pounds off any more successfully than they would on different diets. We don't yet have the foggiest idea what, if any, sway the expansion of sirtfoods to our diet really has on our weight.

Furthermore, will anybody have the option to stay with the dreariness of juices and limit themselves to nourishments on the rundown (and be glad to dump their ordinary cuppa for green tea) for all time? With respect to the features that propose you can appreciate dull chocolate and red wine on this diet – well, truly, it is anything but a green light to devour heaps of either!

Cutting calories will consistently give you results

If you have the funds, the tendency and the stomach for it, I'm very certain it will 'work' somewhat for the time being, if simply because it's a compelling method to limit calories. Also, wine and chocolate aside, the rundown for the most part comprises of the very nourishments dietitians and nutritionists suggest for good wellbeing (think products of the soil!).

Regardless of whether it works all around ok to make it stand separated from the a great many weight-loss designs that have trodden this tired way before likewise is not yet clear. It's reasonable Goggins and Matten will become smash hit diet creators, yet I think the uber bucks will truly stream once the pharmaceutical business figures out how to make sirtuin modulators that we can pop, so there'll be no compelling reason to down one more kale smoothie.

HOW DO SIRTFOOD AND DIET WORKS?

The Sirtfood Diet is developing in ubiquity, however does it truly work for weight loss? Sirtuins are characterized as a bunch of proteins that assume a fundamental job in cell wellbeing and direct different body capacities. These sirtuins may likewise assume a significant job in directing the digestion, fat consuming, expanding bulk and decreasing aggravation. According to sirtfood diet lovers, certain entire nourishments contain sirtfood activators that expansion these proteins in the body. A short rundown of well-known sirtfoods incorporates:

Olive oil

Turmeric

Citrus organic products

Kale

Onions

Buckwheat

Matcha green tea

Parsley

Soy

Pecans

Arugula

Green juice

One significant explanation the sirtfood diet has detonated in ubiquity is because of its stipend of dull chocolate and red wine, as the two things are considered sirtfoods. The case is that by concentrating on these nourishments, fast weight loss will follow without diminishes in bulk. A sirtfood dieter will start their first week drinking green juice made of matcha green tea, lemon juice, parsley, celery, a green apple and arugula three times each week. After the main week, sirtfood dieters come back to eating three suppers for each day made uniquely with sirtfoods and will keep on joining these nourishments all through the rest of the diet.

Does the Sirtfood Diet Actually Work?

There is by all accounts a developing number of famous people and remarkable figures who've touted the sirtfood diet for their ongoing weight loss achievement. Be that as it may, buyers must remember that famous people often approach proficient help when it comes to what they devour and any extra exercise regimens. Also, considers on the adequacy of this diet are thin. Without a doubt, most nourishments recorded are solid entire nourishment alternatives and calorie limitations which are consequently associated with some weight loss. Most of nourishments recorded have mitigating properties, high measures of cancer prevention agents and supplements which are obviously, helpful. Therapeutic specialists caution however, that while snappy weight loss is conceivable on such a diet, a larger part of that underlying loss will be water weight. It might likewise be hazardous for the individuals who take part in moderate to high physical movement.

While regimens like the sirtfood diet still can't seem to be demonstrated when it comes to feasible weight loss, restorative weight loss is a demonstrated and successful answer for any individual who has battled with weight changes and cycles. Diet Demand's primary care physician planned diets are altered to every person for protected, quickened results that lead to long haul achievement.

The most recent diet furor that is slanting among superstars is the sirtfood diet. The diet was brought to the spotlight by two VIP nutritionists in the UK who asserted it as a progressive new diet that works by turning on your "thin quality." according to their case, sirtfood diet can advance quick weight loss, while keeping up bulk and keep you from constant sickness.

How The Diet Works?

These uncommon nourishments initiate sirtuins (SIRTs), a gathering of seven proteins found in the body that manages digestion, irritation and the maturing procedure. These specific proteins are known to shield cells from passing on because of stress. Analysts accept sirtuins additionally improve the body's capacity to consume fat and lift digestion.

Certain plant mixes can build the degree of these proteins in the body. Nourishments containing these mixes are known as "sirtfoods." The Sirtfood diet plan is based around 20 food sources which incorporate kale, red wine, strawberries, onions, soy, parsley, additional virgin olive oil, dull chocolate (85% cocoa), matcha green tea, buckwheat, turmeric, pecans, arugula (rocket), elevated stew, lovage, medjool dates, red chicory, blueberries, escapades, espresso.

Need To Follow The Diet? Here Is How To Do It

The diet is the blend of sirtfoods and calorie limitation to build the degrees of sirtuins in the body. The diet book incorporates feast plans and plans to follow.

It is to be followed in two stages: The underlying stage which goes on for multi week includes limiting calories to 1000kcal for three days. During nowadays you need to drink three sirtfood green juices and one dinner daily that is rich in sirtfoods. During the remainder of the days (four to seven), calorie admission ought to be expanded to 1500kcal. This time you need to expend two sirtfood green juices and two sirtfood-rich dinners daily.

The subsequent stage, otherwise called the support stage, keeps going 14 days. This is where you can see relentless weight loss. During this period, you can eat three adjusted sirtfood-rich dinners consistently, in addition to one green juice. Much after the finish of these stages, the makers of the diet suggest proceeding sirtfoods and green juice into your standard diet.

Alert: There isn't a lot of verification to back this new diet pattern.

There are various craze diets out there. Every one professes to be preferable and progressively viable over the other. If you are attempting to settle on the best diet plan that you can follow, we wager you are befuddled as hellfire. One diet that makes certain to confound you more than some other diet is most likely the Super Carb Diet. Carbs are given a wide compartment by practically all weight watchers. So how might we have a diet on carbs?

The Super Carb Diet was created by Bob Harper, a VIP mentor and host of The Biggest Loser. This diet looks to adjust the admission of proteins and fiber. It does as such by remembering complex starches and negligible fats for the diet. It can assist you with getting in shape adequately without causing you to feel denied.

Super Carb Foods

Nourishments like sweet potatoes, entire grains, lentils, beans, quinoa and couscous contain complex sound carbs. Dissimilar to refined carbs, there complex carbs hold glucose levels under control and actuates weight loss. You can likewise incorporate dark colored rice and cereal to your diet. Butternut squash, beets, cucumber and broccoli are pressed with sound carbs as are natural products like apples, grapes and bananas.

The Super Carb Diet Plan

Right now, need to keep away from entire grains and pasta during lunch and supper. You may have snacks between dinners, yet this can be just organic products or vegetables. To make the diet progressively successful, incorporate ginger, turmeric, garlic and cayenne to your diet. It will invigorate your digestion and lift absorption. Follow this diet for a month and see the difference.

Breakfast: You may have super grains like cereal, quinoa, an English biscuit or an entire grain tortilla for breakfast. Be that as it may, ensure you don't expend in excess of 300 calories.

Lunch and supper: Include boring vegetables and organic products like sweet potatoes, squash, broccoli, apples and grapes to your dinners. Additionally include a segment of protein-rich nourishments like fish and eggs. Vegetarians can add tofu and yogurt to their diet. Ensure you limit your calorie admission to 400 and 500 calories each for lunch and supper individually.

The Super Carb Diet was created by Bob Harper, a superstar coach and host of The Biggest Loser. This diet looks to adjust the admission of proteins and fiber. It does as such by remembering complex sugars and negligible fats for the diet. It can assist you with getting more fit adequately without causing you to feel denied.

Super Carb Foods

Nourishments like sweet potatoes, entire grains, lentils, beans, quinoa and couscous contain complex sound carbs. Not at all like refined carbs, there complex carbs hold glucose levels within proper limits and instigates weight loss. You can likewise incorporate dark colored rice and oats to your diet. Butternut squash, beets, cucumber and broccoli are pressed with sound carbs as are organic products like apples, grapes and bananas.

The Super Carb Diet Plan

Right now, need to maintain a strategic distance from entire grains and pasta during lunch and supper. You may have snacks between suppers, however this can be just organic products or vegetables. To make the diet progressively compelling, incorporate ginger, turmeric, garlic and cayenne to your diet. It will invigorate your digestion and lift absorption. Follow this diet for a month and see the difference.

Breakfast: You may have super grains like oats, quinoa, an English biscuit or an entire grain tortilla for breakfast. In any case, ensure you don't devour in excess of 300 calories.

Lunch and supper: Include bland vegetables and natural products like sweet potatoes, squash, broccoli, apples and grapes to your dinners. Likewise include a segment of protein-rich nourishments like fish and eggs. Vegetarians can add tofu and yogurt to their diet. Ensure you limit your calorie admission to 400 and 500 calories each for lunch and supper separately.

It sounds unrealistic...

If someone educated you concerning a diet that permits you to drink red wine and eat dull chocolate—while likewise shedding kilos like insane—your first inquiry may be: what's the trick?

Yet, evidently there isn't one, according to the makers of the Sirtfood Diet, the most recent weight-loss plan creating a ruckus on the interwebs and getting love on Instagram. That is on the grounds that wine and chocolate, alongside nourishments like strawberries, rocket pecans, and kale, are among an assortment of "Sirtfoods" that supposedly initiate your body's characteristic "thin qualities" to assist you with consuming fat.

It's unmistakable why this diet is so well known (see: wine, chocolate), however is it unrealistic? Here's all that you have to know.

What It Is

The creators of The Sirtfood Diet exhort eating nourishments rich in sirtuins, a sort of plant-based protein that has given some guarantee in clinical investigations to improve metabolic wellbeing. "The eating plan itself is intended to 'turn on' the sirtuin qualities (especially SIRT-1), which are accepted to support digestion, increment fat consuming, battle aggravation, and check hunger," says enrolled dietician, Edwina Clark, head of nourishment and health for Yummly.

Early examinations propose that kilojoule limitation and resveratrol (a polyphenol found in nourishments like grapes, blueberries, and peanuts), actuate the SIRT-1 quality, and these two standards support the Sirtfood way to deal with eating.

The diet endures a sum of three weeks and is isolated into two stages. During stage one, you restrict yourself to three Sirtfood green juices (containing kale, arugula, parsley, celery, green apple, lemon squeeze, and green tea) and one Sirtfood-rich supper every day, totaling around 4000 kilojoules every day, says Dr Caroline Apovian, chief of the Nutrition and Weight Management Center at the Boston Medical Center.

For the following four days, you drink two Sirtfood green squeezes and eat two Sirtfood-rich dinners, which brings your kilojoule aggregate to around 6000 every day.

Stage two, or the upkeep arrange, endures 14 days. During those two weeks, you should have three Sirtfood-rich suppers and one Sirtfood green squeeze day by day.

When those three weeks are up, there's no set intend to follow. To proceed on the Sirtfood way, you should simply change every one of your suppers to incorporate however many Sirtfoods as could be expected under the circumstances. Exercise is additionally supported (30 minutes of movement, five days per week), however getting sweat-soaked isn't the principle focal point of the weight-loss plan.

See probably the craziest diets individuals have really attempted:

Advantages and disadvantages

The Sirtfood Diet incorporates numerous nutritious nourishments that are advantageous for weight loss, for example, celery, kale, green tea, Medjool dates, lean chicken, lean red meat, and parsley, says Apovian. The diet additionally confines or kills numerous nourishments that are known to cause weight increase, for example, refined flours, included sugars, and handled nourishments with practically zero dietary benefit. What's more, because of that absurdly low kilojoule consumption, adherents will probably get in shape gave they stay on track, she says.

"Proof to date proposes that kilojoule limitation and irregular fasting can be a compelling procedure for weight loss and improving metabolic wellbeing," says Clark. "In any case, this may not be fitting for everybody," she says.

The long haul supportability of this arrangement is flawed. When you're past the initial not many weeks, there's no eating procedure to follow other than adding more Sirtfoods to every dinner. This makes the diet substantially more adaptable than most, which is a tremendous advantage, however a three-week extended length of hardship could without much of a stretch lead to indulging during stage two, eventually putting you back at the starting point.

As diets go, one that touts the advantages of red wine and dim chocolate utilization seems like a thick cut of dieting paradise. In any case, that is not everything to the most current U.K. big name diet pattern, the Sirtfood Diet.

The diet was created by creators and sustenance specialists Aidan Goggins and Glen Matten, who both learned at the University of Surrey and hold graduate degrees in healthful drug. In Goggins and Matten's book The Sirtfood Diet, they depict an eating plan that vows to "switch on your 'thin quality,'" or rather a class of qualities that code for sirtuins (SIRTs), which are proteins that help manage fat creation and capacity.

"We became charmed by the potential for specific nourishments to turn on a ground-breaking reusing process in the body that gets out cell waste and consumes fat. They do this by actuating the equivalent 'thin' qualities that are enacted by fasting and exercise. We call these nourishments sirtfoods," Matten says. "When we put these nourishments into an extraordinary Sirtfood Diet and trialed it, members shed seven pounds in seven days and detailed inclination the best they at any point had."

The book was distributed in January 2016 in the U.K. furthermore, Matten hopes to report the U.S. discharge "unavoidably."

The Science of the Sirtfood Diet {brief)

Expending nourishments rich in "sirtuin activators" — including red wine, kale, arugula, buckwheat, apples, blueberries, tricks, red onions, pecans, strawberries, additional virgin olive oil, parsley, dull chocolate, green tea, and espresso among others — should upregulate the outflow of SIRT qualities, expanding the creating sirtuin proteins that will (ideally) hinder the gathering of fat. You've likely known about the most celebrated of the sirtuin activators: Resveratrol, a compound found in red wine.

In 2003, David A. Sinclair, Ph.D., an educator in the Department of Genetics at Harvard Medical School, distributed the consequences of the principal concentrate to propose that resveratrol eases back maturing in a manner like calorie limitation — that is, by animating the SIRT2 quality, which advances DNA soundness, builds the generation of the body's own cancer prevention agents, and slows down fat creation. From that point forward, a lot more sirtuin activators (and the nourishments where they're found) have been identified, and the rundown of potential advantages from expending them continues developing.

Potential Benefits of the Sirtfood Diet

Sirtuins have additionally been attached to the working of the anxious, cardiovascular, and safe frameworks, just as liver, bone, muscle, foundational microorganism, and tissue recovery, according to 2014 article "The Controversial World of Sirtuins" distributed in the diary Drug Discovery Today: Technologies. Sirtuins have additionally been attributed with assisting with battling many age-related illnesses, including malignancy, cardiovascular sickness, metabolic issue, osteoporosis, neurodegenerative ailments, and joint inflammation.

Studies have additionally uncovered that sirtuins can diminish aggravation, hypoxic worry (as may be brought about by poor flow), heat stun, and genotoxic (DNA harming) worry, according to 2011 article "Sirtuins at a Glance" in the Journal of Cell Science, which takes note of that irritation is a significant reason for maturing and maturing related maladies.

Sirtfood Diet at a Glance

The primary period of the diet keeps going multi week. During the underlying three days, members are permitted to devour 1,000 calories as three sirtfood juices and one sirtfood-rich dinner, which can likewise join non-sirtfoods. During days four to seven, calories are expanded to 1,500 every day, and can incorporate two sirtfood juices and two sirtfood-rich suppers.

The subsequent stage keeps going 14 days, and it is during this time most weight loss allegedly happens regardless of a shift away from calorie limitation. The attention is currently on solidifying your new-gained sirtfood dietary patterns with three sirtfood-rich dinners and one green squeeze a day.

SIRTFOOD AND DISEASE

The investigation of maturing in invertebrate model creatures has delivered central new perceptions about instruments of eukaryotic maturing. Among the qualities that have been appeared to direct maturing in different species are SIR2 and its practical orthologs that make up a group of protein deacetylases named Sirtuins. It has been known for four decades that histones can be acetylated (Roth et al., 2001), despite the fact that the catalysts that acetylate and deacetylate lysine buildups on histones and different proteins have just been found all the more as of late. Histone and protein deacetylases fall into four classes with the yeast proteins Rpd3 (class I), Hda1 (class II), and Sir2 (class III) filling in as sanction individuals from the three significant classes (Blander and Guarente, 2004, Sengupta and Seto, 2004). Human HDAC11, the sole individual from class IV, is moderated in mice and D. melanogaster however not C. elegans and yeast (Gao et al., 2002). Class III deacetylases, the Sirtuins, are special in that they require NAD as a cofactor (Blander and Guarente, 2004, Denu, 2003). In an entangled two-advance response, Sirtuins couple lysine deacetylation to NAD hydrolysis, yielding O-acetyl-ADP-ribose and nicotinamide (Denu, 2003). All things considered, Sirtuin action might be constrained by cell [NAD]/[NADH] proportions and reacts to changes in cell digestion (Lin et al., 2000, Lin et al., 2002, Lin et al., 2004).

Both class I and III deacetylases have been connected to maturing (Bitterman et al., 2003), albeit most examinations have concentrated on the class III Sirtuins. Expanded Sir2 action has been accounted for to improve yeast replicative life range (depicted underneath) (Kaeberlein et al., 1999), just as the life length of C. elegans and D. melanogaster (Rogina and Helfand, 2004, Tissenbaum and Guarente, 2001). Conversely, decreased Sir2 action broadens yeast ordered life range (portrayed beneath) under supplement poor conditions or in blend with transformations in qualities, for example, RAS2 and SCH9, which work in glucose-responsive sign transduction pathways (Fabrizio et al., 2005). Various investigations of Sirtuin work have been acted in mammalian cells, in spite of the fact that it stays obscure whether Sirtuins legitimately control life length. Right now, analyze the job of Sir2 and different Sirtuins in invertebrate maturing. Also, we examine Sirtuin works in warm blooded creatures and how they may influence human life span and age-related sickness.

Sirtuins and Yeast Replicative Life Span

The topsy-turvy division normal for the yeast S. cerevisiae is the reason for replicative life-range estimations. Mother cells give ascend by maturing to littler, effectively recognizable girl cells. Micromanipulation is utilized to expel progressive little girls, which are considered ages and arranged (Mortimer and Johnston, 1959). Extensive exertion has been coordinated toward identifying qualities that direct yeast replicative maturing. Analysts have set accentuation on transformations and intercessions that lengthen yeast life range, thinking that mediations diminishing life length may not be straightforwardly connected to the maturing procedure. Until this point, around 50 changes, for the most part quality cancellations, have been accounted for to bring about expanded replicative life range (Bitterman et al., 2003, Kaeberlein et al., 2005b).

The principal interface among SIR2 and maturing originated from the finding that specific transformations in a segment of the yeast SIR complex brought about augmentation of replicative life range (Kennedy et al., 1995). At that point, the SIR complex (Sir2, Sir3, and Sir4) was known to curb interpretation of two yeast quiet mating-type loci (which contain untranscribed duplicates of mating assurance qualities) and of qualities put close to yeast telomeres (Rusche et al., 2003). At first, it was conjectured that SIR movement at telomeres might be managing yeast maturing, however followup examination demonstrated that improved life range corresponded with relocalization of the SIR complex to the nucleolus (Kennedy et al., 1997), the subnuclear area of ribosomal DNA (rDNA) qualities and a significant site of ribosome biogenesis.

Homologous recombination inside rDNA rehashes can prompt the development of extrachromosomal rDNA circles (ERCs). Sir2 hinders rDNA recombination and can likewise quell translation of embedded qualities that are interpreted by PolII (Rusche et al., 2003). Since ERCs contain a site of replication inception however no centromere, they experience replication during S stage yet stay in the mother cell core during mitosis. Aggregation of ERCs inside a mother cell is one reason for yeast replicative maturing (Sinclair and Guarente, 1997). Without SIR2, the pace of ERC arrangement is improved and cells are fleeting (Kaeberlein et al., 1999). Diminished recombination intervened by SIR2 overexpression or cancellation of the FOB1 quality prompts lower ERC levels and results in expanded yeast replicative life length (Defossez et al., 1999, Kaeberlein et al., 1999). Fob1 has replication fork blocking movement and furthermore advances recombination inside the rDNA (Kobayashi and Horiuchi, 1996). Albeit expanded movement of Sir2 orthologs is related with life-range expansion in worms and flies (Rogina and Helfand, 2004, Tissenbaum and Guarente, 2001), there is no proof of a connection among ERCs and maturing in any life form other than yeast.

Calorie Restriction and Yeast Replicative Aging

Calorie limitation (CR), characterized as a decrease in organismal vitality consumption, has been appeared to improve life span of creatures running from yeast to warm blooded animals. Yeast is a significant framework wherein to contemplate calorie limitation since supplement responsive pathways directing cell development are generally surely known. CR in yeast can be initiated by a decrease of glucose in the development media or by transformations, (for example, the erasure of hexokinase 2) that lessen the digestion of glucose (Lin et al., 2000). The job of Sir2 in the calorie limitation reaction is questionable (Guarente, 2005, Kennedy et al., 2005). Significantly, it stays undisputed that expanded Sir2 action prompts replicative life-range augmentation; just the proposed connection among Sir2 and CR has been raised doubt about.

At first, it was accounted for that SIR2 was required forever range augmentation by calorie limitation in yeast. This end depended on an additionally undisputed finding that brief strains lacking SIR2 didn't display life-length expansion under CR conditions. Without SIR2, ERCs aggregate. Along these lines, the finding that CR neglects to expand life length in a strain lacking SIR2 can be deciphered in one of two different ways. Either CR legitimately prompts a decrease in ERC levels by improving Sir2 movement (Lin et al., 2000) or yeast strains lacking SIR2, which have an inexact half decrease in mean replicative life-length potential, rashly capitulate to raised ERCs and don't live long enough to react to CR.

It has been accounted for that CR causes hearty life-length expansion without SIR2 as long as ERCs are kept at low levels by erasure of FOB1 (Kaeberlein et al., 2004), a finding that has since been upheld by another gathering (Lamming et al., 2005) yet not bolstered in a previous investigation utilizing a different yeast strain foundation (Lin et al., 2002). This was deciphered by Kaeberlein et al. to demonstrate that SIR2 is required not as an immediate effector of calorie limitation however in a roundabout way to keep up low ERC levels and along these lines empower the cells to live long enough to react to CR (Kaeberlein et al., 2004). To repeat, there is general understanding that CR can expand replicative life range in a strain lacking both SIR2 and FOB1 however not in a strain that needs just SIR2. Be that as it may, followup examinations and translations thereof have driven different gatherings to different ends with respect to the significance of Sir2 for the CR reaction (see underneath). CR actualized by a decrease in amino acids is likewise answered to broaden yeast replicative life length (Jiang et al., 2002). Expansion right now free of SIR2.

One of the creators (B.K.K.) is at the focal point of the contest with respect to the significance of Sir2 in the CR reaction. Notwithstanding, we will exhibit the two perspectives as well as could be expected. The discussion as of now lays on the degree of glucose restriction used to actualize the CR reaction. Guarente, Lin, Sinclair, and partners accept that lessening the glucose fixation from 2% to 0.5% (4× decrease) is perfect since it minimally affects yeast development rate and might be all the more physiologically like degrees of calorie limitation utilized in other model life forms (Lamming et al., 2006, Lin and Guarente, 2006). They recommend that CR interceded by a decrease in glucose fixation to 0.05% might be SIR2 autonomous and intervened through a different system. Kaeberlein, Kennedy, and partners have to a great extent, however not only, utilized 0.05% glucose (40× decrease) since it amplifies life-length expansion (Kaeberlein et al., 2004, Kaeberlein et al., 2005a, Kaeberlein et al., 2006b), allowing simpler understanding of epistasis examination (Clancy et al., 2002). They bolster a model whereby life-range augmentation by CR is Sirtuin autonomous and not on a very basic level different at either level of glucose constraint (Kaeberlein et al., 2005a, Kaeberlein et al., 2006a, Kaeberlein et al., 2006b). At either 0.5% or 0.05% glucose, CR broadens life length in a way subject to the supplement responsive kinases, TOR, PKA, and SCH9 (the Akt ortholog) (see brief conversation underneath) (Fabrizio et al., 2001, Kaeberlein et al., 2005d, Lin et al., 2000). These supplement responsive kinases control various downstream reactions including ribosome biogenesis and cell development, stress reactions, and autophagy. Which of these are significant forever length augmentation stays to be resolved. Despite the fact that erasure of SCH9 reduces recombination in the rDNA (Prusty and Keil, 2004), it is obvious from an assortment of epistasis contemplates that this phenotype doesn't clarify replicative life-length augmentation. For instance, twofold freaks lacking both SCH9 and FOB1 endure any longer than freaks lacking just FOB1, which as of now have very low degrees of ERCs (Kaeberlein et al., 2005d).

Life-range expansion by CR at 0.5% or 0.05% glucose can happen without SIR2, as long as FOB1 is likewise erased (Kaeberlein et al., 2004, Lamming et al., 2005). Two discoveries drove Lamming et al. to recommend that different Sirtuins were, as one with Sir2, acting in an excess design to intercede the calorie limitation reaction under these conditions (Lamming et al., 2005).

To start with, nicotinamide, a known inhibitor of Sirtuin enzymatic action, can hinder probably a portion of the life-length augmentation by CR even without Sir2 (Kaeberlein et al., 2005a, Lamming et al., 2005). Second, a screen for qualities that when over expressed prompted upgraded rDNA hushing brought about the identification of HST2, another Sirtuin (Lamming et al., 2005). In spite of the fact that Hst2 is regularly cytoplasmic (Perrod et al., 2001), under CR conditions it is accounted for to relocalize to the core (Lamming et al., 2005). Further, Lamming et al. report that, comparably to strains lacking SIR2, yeast lacking just HST2 display raised rDNA recombination and a short life range. The discovering in regards to rDNA recombination appears differently in relation to a past report by Gasser and associates, who found that a yeast strain lacking HST2 shows decreased rDNA recombination (Perrod et al., 2001).

At 0.5% glucose, Lamming et al. report that CR neglects to expand life range in a strain lacking both SIR2 and HST2, prompting the end that CR broadens life length by lessening rDNA recombination and ERC development in a SIR2-and HST2-subordinate design (Lamming et al., 2005). Hst1, another Sirtuin, may

68

likewise make up for Sir2 in certain strains. Another gathering has discovered utilizing the equivalent hereditary foundation that CR broadens life range in yeast strains that need SIR2, HST2, and FOB1 or in yeast that additionally need HST1 (Kaeberlein et al., 2006b). The reason(s) for these divergent discoveries are as a rule effectively discussed (Kaeberlein et al., 2006b, Lamming et al., 2006).

At long last, life span expansion by CR has been connected to cell breath. Work from Guarente, Sinclair, and partners has prompted the model that CR prompts raised NAD levels (Lin et al., 2002), decreased NADH levels (Lin et al., 2004), as well as diminished nicotinamide levels (Anderson et al., 2003, Bitterman et al., 2002), which thus lead to Sir2 enactment. Decreasing glucose levels in yeast improves the respiratory pace of the facultative anaerobe, and it has been suggested this upgraded pace of breath prompts expanded [NAD]/[NADH] proportions. Besides, CR neglects to increment replicative life range of respiratory-insufficient yeast (Lin et al., 2002), in spite of the fact that this finding has additionally been questioned (Kaeberlein et al., 2005a). Regardless of whether differential degrees of glucose hardship underlie the divergent discoveries of these examinations likewise keeps on being discussed (Kaeberlein et al., 2006a, Lin and Guarente, 2006).

Sir2 and Yeast Chronological Life Span

The ordered life-length model maturing in the common habitat since it is a proportion of the endurance of yeast populaces in a nondividing state (Longo et al., 1997). The middle sequential life length of S. cerevisiae wild-type DBY746 or SP1 yeast developed in glucose medium (SDC) is 6 to 7 days. Under these conditions wild-type DBY746 cells have overabundance ethanol accessible for vitality creation and keep up high metabolic rates for most of the life length. A type of serious calorie limitation, accomplished by changing cells from ethanol/glucose-containing medium to water between days 1 and 5, causes a reduction in metabolic rates and stretches out endurance by 2-to 3-overlay (Fabrizio et al., 2004a, Longo et al., 1997).

Yeast strains with decreased movement of Ras2 or any of the supplement responsive kinases Sch9, PKA, and TOR have broadened sequential life length (Fabrizio et al., 2001, Fabrizio et al., 2003, Fabrizio et al., 2004b, Powers et al., 2006). Significantly, Sch9 is an utilitarian homolog of Akt/PKB, a part of the moderated master maturing pathways of worms, flies, and mice (Longo and Finch, 2003).

As opposed to the job of ERCs in yeast replicative maturing, superoxide seems to assume a focal job in S. cerevisiae sequential maturing and demise. Truth be told, the superoxide-delicate 4Fe-4S group catalyst aconitase is inactivated going before the high mortality stage (Fabrizio et al., 2001), and overexpression of the superoxide dismutases SOD1 or SOD2 expands ordered life range (Fabrizio et al., 2003). Unconstrained DNA transformation recurrence likewise increments with sequential age, in spite of the fact that its job in maturing and demise remains inadequately comprehended (Fabrizio et al., 2004a, Fabrizio et al., 2005).

The job of Sir2 in the ordered endurance of nondividing yeast cells has as of late been inspected (Fabrizio et al., 2005) and gives off an impression of being very different from its job in the yeast replicative life range. Cancellation of SIR2 expands pressure opposition yet has no impact on the sequential life length of wild-type yeast developed and kept up in medium. In any case, erasure of SIR2 expands further the ordered life length brought about by serious CR (hatching in water) (Fabrizio et al., 2005) or brought about by transformations that abatement PKA or Sch9 action. Besides, the overexpression of SIR2 has no impact on the ordered life length of wild-type cells and lessens the life range of cells lacking Sch9 action (Fabrizio et al., 2005). Different Sirtuins have not been analyzed right now. Proof exists for two potential components by which erasure of SIR2 brings about life-range augmentation when combined with diminished supplement responsive kinase action or CR. To start with, cancellation of SIR2 in blend with diminished PKA or Sch9 movement was found to build the statement of many pressure opposition and sporulation qualities and to diminish the pace of DNA transformations that amass with age in post mitotic conditions (Fabrizio et al., 2005). This stands out from the job of Sir2 in mitotically dynamic cells, where it advances genome security by curbing recombination (Blander and Guarente, 2004). Second, Fabrizio et al. report that cells lacking SIR2 have raised degrees of the liquor dehydrogenase Adh2 (Fabrizio et al., 2005). Mitotically dynamic yeast cells fundamentally create vitality through aging, which prompts the generation of ethanol. As fermentable carbon sources become rare and ethanol aggregates, yeast experience a metabolic shift and start to use ethanol as a vitality source, just entering stationary stage after ethanol levels are generally exhausted. Without Sir2, expanded liquor dehydrogenase action prompts increasingly quick ethanol debasement and section into a progressively steady post mitotic state. The component by which Sir2 contrarily manages Adh2 levels as cells enter a post mitotic state is yet to be resolved. Expanded ethanol take-up may speak to an endeavor by cells lacking SIR2 to get ready for extensive stretches of starvation.

In rundown, despite the fact that the cancellation of SIR2 diminishes and its overexpression expands the yeast replicative life range, changing Sir2 levels doesn't significantly influence the sequential life length. In any case, when joined with serious CR-or life-length expanding changes that diminish the movement of the Ras and Sch9 pathways, transformations in SIR2 do broaden the ordered life range and Sir2 overexpression limits life-length expansion in freaks lacking SCH9. Loss of SIR2 may advance passage into an express that secures cells against maturing during starvation. These outcomes propose that Sir2 assumes totally different jobs in the guideline of replicative and sequential life range.

One Model Organism, Two Measures of Aging?

The replicative life length of yeast is in numerous regards similar to the replicative life range of mammalian fibroblasts and lymphocytes, which experience a set number of populace doublings in culture. Along these lines, replicative maturing in yeast might be a model to consider replicative maturing in mitotically dynamic mammalian cells. Paradoxically, sequential maturing in yeast may serve to display maturing in post mitotic mammalian cells (e.g., neurons) and living beings. Whatever degree do comparative pathways control the systems that lead to replicative and ordered maturing in a similar model living being?

Though prior investigations demonstrated likenesses yet additionally significant differences between the guideline of replicative and ordered life range, later examinations are starting to recommend that there might be just one type of "maturing" in S. cerevisiae with two different ways to quantify it. An enormous scale scan for freaks with an all-inclusive replicative life length prompted the identification of erasure freaks in sch9 and tor1, additionally ensnared in ordered life-range expansion (Fabrizio et al., 2001, Kaeberlein et al., 2005d, Powers et al., 2006). In this manner, supplement responsive kinases control maturing of both mitotic and post mitotic cells. Regardless of whether the effectors that controls each sort of maturing downstream of these kinases are a similar stays to be resolved.

Strikingly, diminished movement of orthologs of these kinases as well as of the pathways where they work lead to life-range expansion in worms, flies, and warm blooded creatures (Kenyon, 2005, Longo and Finch, 2003). We presume that hindrance of these supplement responsive kinases prompts life-length augmentation in warm blooded creatures since it gives particular, helpful impacts in both mitotic and post mitotic populaces of cells. Backing for this originates from yeast replicative and sequential life-range considers yet in addition from life span tests in C. elegans, where it was indicated that diminished insulin/IGF-1 flagging can slow an assortment of age-related phenotypes in particular tissues (Garigan et al., 2002). Comparable impacts have been watched for CR in mice.

For yeast replicative life range, twofold freaks lacking FOB1 and either SCH9 or TOR1 are very seemingly perpetual, proposing that the collection of ERCs brought about by Fob1 may, to a certain extent, veil the impact of loss of SCH9 or TOR1 on replicative life-length augmentation. Hence, ERCs might be liable for one error between the impact of Sir2 on replicative and sequential life range. If Sir2 is missing, ERCs aggregate early and either execute the cell or forestall its division. If Sir2 is over expressed, ERC levels are diminished and replicative life range is upgraded. ERCs may then be seen as an operator that hurries demise specifically in yeast and clouds other progressively widespread maturing forms. Be that as it may, cancellation of SIR2 doesn't expand the replicative life range of strains lacking SCH9 or TOR1 even without FOB1, so there must be other fundamental differences also.

The power of common choice against the presence of "abandons" is extremely high in youthful living beings, yet it decreases at cutting edge ages. Yeast mother cells don't have to create 25 girls to guarantee state endurance or even a maximal settlement development rate, and, therefore, injurious occasions that are specific to old mother cells, (for example, ERC arrangement or diminished development rates) may not be dependent upon counter-selection. Along these lines, ERCs seem, by all accounts, to be a significant reason for maturing just in yeast exposed to conditions not ordinarily experienced in indigenous habitats. Conversely, different instruments of maturing might be moderated, and proof not just from yeast ordered and replicative maturing examines, yet in addition from higher eukaryotes, is starting to show that the Sch9 (Akt), Ras, and Tor might be all inclusive controllers of these systems. Sir2 is obviously significant forever length guideline however it might play either an ace or an enemy of maturing job in different life forms relying upon the accessibility of supplements and on the movement of glucose flagging pathways.

Sir2 and Aging in Other Invertebrates

Two other model life forms where maturing has been contemplated broadly are C. elegans and D. melanogaster. Right now condense discoveries with respect to the job of Sir2 orthologs in maturing in these spineless creatures. Different Sirtuins are available in the two life forms, yet their jobs in maturing have not been learned. In C. elegans, expanded measurement of the SIR2 ortholog, sir-2.1, builds the mean life range by up to half (Tissenbaum and Guarente, 2001), and this augmentation requires the FOXO translation factor DAF-16, which is known to be controlled by the insulin/IGF-1 pathway. Instead of acting legitimately in the insulin/IGF-1 flagging pathway, two late investigations recommend that SIR-2.1 may act in an equal pathway that unites at the purpose of DAF-16 guideline (Wang et al., 2006) (Berdichevsky et al., 2006). In the two examinations, both C. elegans 14-3-3 proteins were identified as SIR-2.1 interactors, a fascinating discovering on the grounds that mammalian 14-3-3 proteins are known to tie FOXO translation factors and sequester them in the cytoplasm (Brunet et al., 1999). In spite of the fact that life-length expansion by SIR-2.1 overexpression can be obstructed by lessening articulation of 14-3-3 proteins, this isn't the situation for transformations that upset the insulin pathway (Wang et al., 2006) (Berdichevsky et al., 2006). For example, the long life length of a daf-2 freak isn't influenced by a decrease in 14-3-3. Indeed, erasure of sir-2.1 doesn't decrease the life range of a daf-2 freak and rather appears to somewhat expand it, steady with the more extended ordered life length watched for yeast lacking both SIR2 and the Akt homolog SCH9 (Berdichevsky et al., 2006, Fabrizio et al., 2005, Wang and Tissenbaum, 2006).

Berdichevsky et al. suggest that SIR-2.1 is a piece of a pressure reaction pathway that manages DAF-16 action in a way reliant on 14-3-3 proteins (Berdichevsky et al., 2006). Steady with this thought, an invalid freak of C. elegans sir-2.1 has a somewhat shorter life length as well as shows affectability to an assortment of stresses including hydrogen peroxide, UV light, and warmth stun (Wang and Tissenbaum, 2006). These outcomes just incompletely concur with those watched for nondividing yeast. Truth be told, in yeast lacking SIR2 the ordered life range is either ordinary or somewhat shorter, DNA transformations are progressively visit, yet affectability to warm stun and oxidative pressure is diminished (Fabrizio et al., 2005). SIR-2.1 is likewise answered to be significant for hushing of transgenes embedded into genomic rehash components, maybe in a way practically equivalent to Sir2-subordinate quieting in yeast (Jedrusik and Schulze, 2003). Regardless of whether this action is significant for life span guideline stays to be resolved.

Different measures have been proposed for calorie limitation in C. elegans, including utilization of eat-2 freaks that eat not exactly wild-type worms, development in axenic media that comes up short on a bacterial nourishment source, and decreased presentation to nourishment source or dietary limitation (Walker et al., 2005). The reliance of sir-2.1 has been resolved for eat-2 freaks and dietary limitation, with to some degree different outcomes. Life-length augmentation by eat-2 freaks is halfway smothered by cancellation of sir-2.1 (Wang and Tissenbaum, 2006). Interestingly, life-length expansion by dietary limitation isn't influenced by sir-2.1 cancellation (M. Kaeberlein, individual correspondence). Likewise, while life-range expansion by sir-2.1 overexpression is daf-16 ward (Tissenbaum and Guarente, 2001), life-length augmentation by CR isn't (Lakowski and Hekimi, 1998).

Little atom activators and inhibitors of Sirtuins have been accounted for. Resveratrol has been proposed as a little atom agonist of yeast Sir2 and of its orthologs in worms, flies, and vertebrates and has been examined

80

with regards to life span (Wood et al., 2004). Resveratrol was identified in a screen for Sirtuin activators utilizing a nonbiological substrate reasonable for high-throughput fluorescent examination (Howitz et al., 2003). In any case, different gatherings have demonstrated that the stimulatory impacts of resveratrol on Sirtuin catalyst enactment are specific to this nonnative substrate (Borra et al., 2005, Kaeberlein et al., 2005c). No improvement of catalyst movement was seen with local acetylated peptides. One plausibility is that resveratrol just invigorates Sirtuin movement toward specific substrates in vivo. On the other hand, the impacts of reseveratrol might be to a great extent Sirtuin autonomous, an attestation predictable with perceptions that the polyphenol compound has a plenty of different exercises. Reports strife about whether resveratrol broadens yeast life range (Howitz et al., 2003, Kaeberlein et al., 2005c).

In C. elegans, sir-2.1-subordinate life-length expansion has been watched for resveratrol (Wood et al., 2004). An ongoing report anyway has recommended that, as opposed to upgrade SIR-2.1 action in worms, resveratrol may expand life range by alienating it (Viswanathan et al., 2005). Likewise, not at all like sir-

2.1 overexpression, resveratrol expands life length in a daf-16-autonomous way. The key objective forever length expansion due to resveratrol treatment seems, by all accounts, to be abu-11, an endoplasmic reticulum (ER) stress-family quality. Either expansion of resveratrol or, inquisitively, sir-2.1 cancellation prompts upgraded abu-11 articulation, which is thusly required forever length augmentation. The creators set forth a model to clarify these apparently confusing discoveries by suggesting that (1) resveratrol may tie to SIR-2.1 and change its specificity toward substrates to such an extent that deacetylation of certain substrates might be upgraded while deacetylation of different substrates is hindered and (2) SIR-2.1 has numerous capacities that encroach on life span guideline with the net impact being that overexpression expands life length. Subsequently, as with Sir2 in yeast, SIR-2.1 in worms may have a few exercises that advance life span and others that breaking points it. Maybe the most intriguing finding from this investigation is that overexpression of abu-11 expands worm life length, ensnaring ER worry as a constraining variable in worm life span.

In flies, the Sir2 ortholog dSir2 has been accounted for to expand life range also (Rogina and Helfand, 2004). What's more, life-length augmentation by CR is obstructed in strains lacking dSir2. These discoveries propose that CR works through a Sir2-subordinate system right now. Freak flies with diminished Rpd3 (class I deacetylases) movement show expanded life length that is subject to dSir2, demonstrating that the two deacetylases are in a solitary pathway managing maturing with Rpd3 upstream (Rogina and Helfand, 2004, Rogina et al., 2002). It has not been resolved whether Rpd3 directs [NAD]/[NADH] proportions in flies. Life-range augmentation by resveratrol is likewise answered to be dSir2 subordinate (Wood et al., 2004). Little is thought about dSir2 work in flies, particularly with respect to maturing specific capacities. This deacetylase has been accounted for to be engaged with transcriptional restraint (Newman et al., 2002), at any rate to some extent through communications with Hairy, a translation calculates included formative guideline (Rosenberg and Parkhurst, 2002). Regardless of whether dSir2 manages the insulin pathway in flies stays to be resolved.

In outline, overexpression of Sir2 orthologs builds fly and worm life range, and the connections between Sir2 orthologs and calorie limitation seem conflicting among living beings and stay to be completely comprehended. It appears to be incomprehensible that the catalyst for analyzing the life range of worms and flies over expressing their Sir2 orthologs got from yeast replicative maturing contemplates, given that the proposed job of Sir2 in life span guideline, lessening ERC generation, appears not to be preserved. We offer three potential clarifications to determine this conundrum. Initially, Sir2 in yeast may have different capacities beside decreased ERC creation that advance replicative life span, and this movement might be rationed. Second, worm and fly Sir2 orthologs may expand life length by stifling recombination at other chromosomal areas that are increasingly delicate (e.g., dreary DNA) and that don't exist in yeast or impact yeast life range. It is difficult to decipher this model with regards to C. elegans where daf-16 is required for the life span impacts of sir-2.1 overexpression. At last, Sir2 orthologs may have developed to couple metabolic signs to specific life span upgrading capacities in different living beings, a model advanced by Guarente and associates (Guarente and Picard, 2005). How this last model would fit with developmental hypotheses of maturing stays to be settled. We should anticipate further trials in every one of these life forms to start to differentiate between these models, or devise a different one. Further adding to the disjointedness is the finding that loss of SIR2 in certain settings improves yeast ordered life length and that its overexpression doesn't influence or lessens sequential life span (Fabrizio et al., 2005).

Sirtuins in Mammals

The maturing phenotype of mice overexpressing Sirt1, and the impacts of CR on life span in a mouse lacking Sirt1, has not yet been resolved. Albeit a dominant part of Sirt1 invalid creatures surrender to formative deformities during early postnatal improvement (Cheng et al., 2003, McBurney et al., 2003), the rest of the mice endure and have phenotypes looking like mice overexpressing IGFBP-1 or lacking IGF-I (Longo and Finch, 2003) (see beneath). In Sirt1-insufficient grown-up survivors, Chen et al. report that calorie limitation neglects to prompt expanded physical movement (Chen et al., 2005a), a typical CR-initiated conduct change in wild-type mice. Be that as it may, physiologic changes like those brought about by CR, for example, decreased blood glucose, triglycerides, and insulin levels, happen ordinarily in these creatures. Despite the fact that these last phenotypes may be relied upon to broaden life span, the impact of Sirt1 inadequacy alone or in blend with CR stays to be set up. By and by, various investigations have announced in well evolved creatures interesting elements of Sirtuins that may relate to maturing. In the accompanying segments, we layout a portion of these discoveries, concentrating on results that identify with maturing and age-related malady.

Sir2/Sirt1, Genomic Instability, and Oncogenesis

Starting connections between Sir2 work and the reaction to DNA harm originated from considers in S. cerevisiae. In proliferating yeast, a few reports demonstrate that Sir2 ensures against DNA harm by inciting nonhomologous end joining and homologous recombination pathways, a capacity which seems to rely upon the derepression of quiet mating-type qualities (Fabrizio et al., 2005, Lee et al., 1999). Sir2 likewise intercedes the deviated legacy of oxidatively harmed proteins during cell division (Aguilaniu et al., 2003).

Mother cells have a constrained life length, however the provinces they produce will keep proliferating as long as adequate supplements are accessible. This hilter kilter legacy limits harmed proteins to the mother cell, likely guaranteeing the age of moderately harm free little girls and proceeded with state proliferation. Interestingly, Sir2 seems to advance ordered age-subordinate genomic unsteadiness in extensive freaks. S. cerevisiae cells aggregate unconstrained DNA transformations with ordered age, and this gathering is radically diminished in strains lacking both SCH9 and SIR2 (Fabrizio et al., 2005). In spite of the fact that this impact of Sir2 insufficiency gives off an impression of being autonomous of the derepression of quiet mating-type qualities, the instruments by which Sir2 advances age-subordinate genomic flimsiness are not known.

In warm blooded creatures, extensive proof exists to recommend that the tumor silencer p53 is an objective for deacetylation by Sirt1 (Cheng et al., 2003). Under typical cell conditions for proliferation, p53, a transcriptional activator, is exceptionally precarious (Gu et al., 2004). p53 adjustment happens as a major aspect of a checkpoint reaction to cell stress (counting DNA harm) and results in proliferative capture, trailed by either reemergence into the cell cycle, senescence, or apoptosis. Acetylation of p53 prompts improved transcriptional enactment as a major aspect of the checkpoint reaction. By deacetylating p53, Sirt1 may kill p53 after recuperation from worry to permit cell proliferation to continue. Despite the fact that it has been indicated that expanded Sirt1 movement prompts hypoacetylation of p53 and constraint of p53 target qualities (Luo et al., 2001, Vaziri et al., 2001), the cell outcomes of this stay being referred to. While Sirt1 movement was initially answered to hinder apoptosis through deacetylation of p53 (Langley et al., 2002, Luo et al., 2001), later reports propose that despite the fact that Sirt1 can deacetylate p53 there is little impact on p53-interceded organic results (Kamel et al., 2006, Solomon et al., 2006). Different pressure reaction related proteins connected to Sirt1 are Ku70 and NF-κB (see underneath) (Cohen et al., 2004, Yeung et al., 2004). Ku70, a DNA fix factor, is accounted for to be an objective for deacetylation by Sirt1, which is another instrument by which Sirt1 may repress cell demise (Cohen et al., 2004).

Developing connections between Sir.2-1 and daf-16 in worms, a few examinations have tried the theory that

Sirt1 can manage mammalian FOXO translation factors through direct authoritative or potentially deacetylation. Sirt1 deacetylation can either prompt actuation or constraint of FOXO-subordinate interpretation relying upon the unique situation (Greer and Brunet, 2005). Current reasoning is that deacetylation of FOXO factors by Sirt1 may prompt enactment of a lot of pressure safe variables, influencing the equalization toward stress opposition and away from apoptosis (Brunet et al., 2004). There additionally exists a mind boggling interchange between FOXOs, Sirt1, and p53, with each having the option to direct the other two in probably some cell settings (Greer and Brunet, 2005). Since every one of the three of these proteins has been connected to maturing, it is basic that future investigations outline these mind boggling cooperations.

Sirt1 work has likewise been inspected with regards to cell senescence in cell culture. Chua et al. reports that mouse undeveloped organism fibroblasts lacking Sirt1 are impervious to senescence within the sight of sublethal, incessant oxidative pressure (Chua et al., 2005). Strangely, oncogene-instigated senescence happens ordinarily in these cells. Reliable with this outcome, nicotinamide, a sirtuin inhibitor, has been accounted for in another examination to expand the replicative life range of essential human fibroblasts (Lim et al., 2006), albeit no trials were exhibited that straightforwardly connect the activities of nicotinamide to Sirt1 or different Sirtuins right now. Primer investigations inspecting joins between Sirt1 capacity and malignant growth recommend that it is improved Sirt1 movement that might be oncogenic. For example, treatment of human bosom and lung malignancy cells with Sirtinol, another Sirt1 inhibitor, has been found to prompt a senescent-like development capture (Ota et al., 2006). Related discoveries were accounted for by Ford et al. (Portage et al., 2005), who utilized RNAi to quiet articulation of Sirt1. Right now, decrease of Sirt1 prompted development capture as well as apoptosis in human epithelial malignant growth lines yet not essential epithelial cells.

Inhibitors of class I and class II histone deacetylases are under clinical preliminaries as chemotherapeutic specialists. The antitumor impacts of these inhibitors likely originate from their capacity to reactivate translation of tumor silencer qualities in blend with DNA-demethylating operators. A comparable job has as of late been proposed for the Sirt1 inhibitors, which were found to advance the reactivation of tumor silencer quality interpretation in human bosom and colon malignant growth lines (Pruitt et al., 2006). Right now, articulation could be accomplished without inhibitors of DNA methylation despite the fact that the advertisers being referred to remained exceptionally methylated. In spite of the fact that there is no broad understanding concerning the systems by which Sirt1 may advance oncogenesis, these examinations by and large point to the requirement for additional examination and the potential job of Sirtuin inhibitors in disease treatment. These outcomes might be reliable with the impact of SIR2 cancellation transformations in expanding protection from oxidative harm, decreasing DNA harm, and broadening the yeast ordered life length in mix with changes in supplement responsive kinases (Fabrizio et al., 2005). In this way, both yeast Sir2 and mammalian Sirt1 can advance DNA harm or oncogenesis, despite the fact that they likewise assume significant jobs in ensuring against harm during cell development and organismal improvement.

Less firmly identified with the different Sirtuins, the essential movement of Sirt6 is ADP-ribosylation instead of deacetylation (Liszt et al., 2005). An ongoing report finds that mice lacking Sirt6 display upgraded genome precariousness prompting a wide scope of chromosomal inconsistencies just as phenotypes looking like untimely maturing, including cachexia, kyphosis, and osteopenia (Mostoslavsky et al., 2006). Numerous different changes prompting progeria in well evolved creatures are related with genome shakiness. Mostoslavsky et al. find that mice lacking Sirt6 have a scope of sensitivities to DNA-harming operators including MMS and ionizing radiation that are steady with absconds in base extraction fix (Mostoslavsky et al., 2006). The specific job of Sirt6 right now stays to be resolved.

Sirtuins and Mammalian Metabolism

Diminished insulin/IGF-I flagging is personally connected to improved life span in worms, flies, and mice (Longo and Finch, 2003). Further, cancellation of the yeast orthologs of Akt and Ras, which work downstream of mammalian insulin/IGF-I, brings about broadened replicative and sequential life length in yeast (Fabrizio et al., 2001, Fabrizio et al., 2003, Fabrizio et al., 2004b, Lin et al., 2000). Since insulin flagging connections extracellular glucose levels to cell digestion, and expanded life length in worms overexpressing sir-

2.1 is reliant on daf-16, extensive exertion has been given to revealing the associations between Sirt1 capacity and digestion in well evolved creatures. Until this point in time, the aftereffects of these examinations have not created an away from of the job of Sirt1 in these procedures.

Two examinations have analyzed the capacity of Sirt1 in the arrival of insulin by pancreatic β cells. Bordone et al. revealed that a siRNA-upheld decrease of Sirt1 articulation in β cell lines prompts an expansion in the statement of uncoupling protein 2 (UCP2) and a decrease in insulin emission (Bordone et al., 2006). This finding may phenocopy nourishment hardship, which is known to actuate UCP2 articulation and diminish insulin discharge. In a subsequent report, Sirt1 articulation was raised specifically in the mouse pancreas, prompting decreased UCP2 articulation and upgraded insulin discharge during glucose incitement (Moynihan et al., 2005). Sirt1 additionally initiates gluconeogenic qualities and hepatic glucose yield through the transcriptional coactivator PGC-1 α (Rodgers et al., 2005). At any rate as to β cell work, decreased Sirt1 may impersonate as opposed to hinder the impacts of either CR or low-plasma IGF-I, in concurrence with different phenotypes portrayed underneath for Sirt1 invalid mice, including little body size and expanded degrees of IGFBP-1.

Sirtuins additionally have works in fat tissue. For example, Picard et al. show that Sirt1 advances fat activation in mammalian adipocytes by stifling PPARγ (Picard et al., 2004), and decreased fat substance has been connected to expanded life span (Bluher et al., 2003). Nonetheless, it is capacity and not the preparation of fat that has been reliably connected with life span expansion in worms, flies, and mice, evidently as a feature of a program planned for enduring extensive stretches of starvation (Longo and Finch, 2003). Remarkably Sirt3, a mitochondrial Sirtuin, is communicated to a great extent in darker fat, proposing a job for this deacetylase in versatile thermogenesis (Shi et al., 2005). Connections among maturing and Sirt3 presently can't seem to be accounted for.

Are the metabolic outcomes of adjusting Sirt1 levels professional or against maturing (or both)? Raised Sirt1 articulation may broaden life range by diminishing fat stockpiling. Then again, decreased Sirt1 levels cause changes undifferentiated from those saw in the enduring IGF-I-insufficient mice (McBurney et al., 2003). The job for Sirt1 in decreasing the statement of the IGF restricting protein, IGFBP-1, in expanding hepatic glucose yield, in expanding pancreatic insulin discharge, in activating fat, and in forestalling a smaller person phenotype raises the likelihood that Sirt1 may play both a master and hostile to maturing job in warm blooded creatures as has been appeared in S. cerevisiae, C. elegans, and mammalian cells (Fabrizio et al., 2005, Kaeberlein et al., 1999).

It will be imperative to decide if the job of Sirt1 in diminishing IGFBP-1 and fat stockpiling and expanding hepatic glucose yield and pancreatic insulin emission is proof for passage into a genius maturing mode and additionally whether Sirt1 controls frameworks that may advance physical action during times of starvation to discover nourishment or staying away from predation. Truth be told, the expansion in movement of mice during CR requires Sirt1 (Chen et al., 2005a). One plausibility is that, during CR, mammalian Sirt1 assumes a job in hindering section into a non-reproductive and decreased physical movement stage that might be portrayed by a more slow maturing rate (McBurney et al., 2003, Chen et al., 2005a), as appeared for the job of Sir2 in the S. cerevisiae sequential life range (Fabrizio et al., 2005).

Sirtuins and Neuro-degeneration

Both in C. elegans and well evolved creatures, specific neurological capacities have been ascribed to Sir2 orthologs. To consider neuronal cytotixicity in worms, Parker et al. built up a framework in which a part of the human Huntington infection related protein, htt, is communicated in contact receptor neurons (Parker et al., 2005). Either expanded measurements of sir-2.1 or introduction to resveratrol saved neuronal brokenness. The creators conjectured that SIR-2.1-subordinate enactment of stress-responsive daf-16 targets might be advancing cell endurance. Nothing to date has been accounted for that straightforwardly connects Sirt1 with htt in warm blooded creatures. Be that as it may, Sirt1 appears to repress axonal degeneration, a procedure that often goes before neuronal passing in neurodegenerative infections, for example, Parkinson's and Alzheimer's (Araki et al., 2004). This action of Sirt1 was found in light of the fact that moderate axonal degeneration in a strain of freak mice was connected to overexpression of a NAD biosynthetic compound. Of note, another exquisite investigation looking at axonal degeneration credited the advantages of expanded NAD biosynthesis to Sirt1-free modifications in neighborhood bioenergetics (Wang et al., 2005). These creators pinpointed the deteriorative decrease in NAD levels to axons and not the core where Sirt1 action is probably managed. A last report identified with neuro-degeneration analyzed NF-κB motioning in microglia, an action connected to amyloid-β neuronal demise and Alzheimer's ailment, finding that overexpression of Sirt1 curbed NF-κB motioning by lessening RelA/p65 acetylation (Chen et al., 2005b). Together, these discoveries call for expanded assessment of Sirt1 as a potential defensive operator in neurons.

Sir2 Deacetylases: Anti-maturing, Pro-maturing, or Both?

In outline, the outcomes in S. cerevisiae and invertebrate model frameworks, combined with likenesses between Sirt1-insufficient and extensive IGF-I-lacking smaller person mice (Longo and Finch, 2003), propose that the most secure wager now is that Sir2 deacetylases play both ace and hostile to maturing jobs in different settings. One speculation to be tried is that decreased Sir2/Sirt1 movement can advance life-range expansion by causing section into a moderate maturing

97

starvation reaction stage though Sir2/Sirt1 overexpression can advance life-length augmentation by actuating different changes, for example, fat breakdown and improved physical action.

The field basically anticipates investigations of mouse life span. Will mice overexpressing Sirt1, mice insufficient in Sirt1, or neither appreciate broadened life span? Will CR expand life length in mice lacking Sirt1? Will Sirt1 lack further expand the life range of mice with transformations in the IGF-1/Akt pathway? Other basic robotic inquiries additionally stay to be replied. What are the key focuses of the Sirt1 deacetylase? Does resveratrol invigorate Sirtuin action toward natural substrates and, if things being what they are, which ones? These outcomes and others will no uncertainty start to clarify the connections among Sirtuins and mammalian life span.

Over the previous decade, MIT researcher Leonard Guarente '74 and others have indicated that low-calorie diets incite a complete physiological reaction that advances endurance, all arranged by a lot of proteins called sirtuins.

Presently, Guarente and partners have indicated that sirtuins are additionally liable to assume a key job in the mental reaction to dietary limitation. When sirtuins are raised in the cerebrum, as happens when nourishment admission is cut, serotonin levels drop in mice and the creatures become substantially more on edge. Besides, in two huge hereditary investigations of people, the group found that changes that lift creation of sirtuins are usually connected with higher paces of nervousness and frenzy issue.

The specialists accept this nervousness might be a developmental adjustment that makes creatures— including people—increasingly careful under the pressure of scavenging all the more broadly for rare nourishment.

"It bodes well, in light of the fact that social impacts would be as versatile, and as chose by advancement, as physiological impacts," says -Guarente, an educator of science. "I don't believe it's amazing that conduct truly falls under the umbrella of common choice."

Guarente found around 20 years back that sirtuins drag out life range in yeast; from that point forward, they have been appeared to have comparative impacts in worms, mice, and different creatures. Ordinarily turned on in light of stresses, for example, starvation or aggravation, the mixes coordinate an assortment of hormonal networks, administrative proteins, and qualities, with a net impact of keeping cells alive and solid.

His new research, distributed online in Cell in December, inspected mice with raised degrees of the SIRT1 protein in their cerebrums and mice with no SIRT1. Scientists set them on a round raised stage with two quadrants secured by a divider and two unprotected quadrants. "Ordinary mice will invest a lot of energy wandering out into the unprotected district, and super-restless mice will in general remain in the ensured zone," Guarente says.

The mice with extremely high sirtuin levels invested substantially more energy closer to the dividers, proposing that they were progressively restless. Mice lacking sirtuin were considerably more bold.

The group researched the cell instrument behind this wonder. They found that sirtuins help control levels of the synapse serotonin, since quite a while ago known to be basic for state of mind guideline.

The new research recommends that nervousness could be treated with drugs that hinder sirtuins. Be that as it may, it additionally offers purpose behind alert when treating patients with drugs that initiate sirtuins, a few of which are presently in clinical preliminaries for diabetes and other metabolic ailments. Those medications can't enter the cerebrum, however a few specialists are investigating the probability of utilizing sirtuin activators to treat neurological issue, for example, Alzheimer's malady. If such medications were created and affirmed, specialists may need to look for tension as a potential symptom.

"We need to learn as much as we can about the science of sirtuins, to illuminate the utilization regarding sirtuin medications to treat ailments," Guarente says. "The more we think about the science, the better position we'll be in to realize how to utilize the medications, how to portion them, and how to envision any conceivable symptoms."

SUPERFOODS

Healthfully, there is nothing of the sort as a super food.

The term was instituted for showcasing purposes to impact nourishment patterns and sell items.

The nourishment business offers the super food name on supplement rich food sources with an alleged ability to decidedly influence wellbeing.

Despite the fact that numerous nourishments could be depicted as super, it's imperative to comprehend that there is no single nourishment that holds the way to great wellbeing or infection counteraction.

Be that as it may, since the expression "super food" doesn't appear to be going anyplace at any point in the near future, it might merit investigating some sound alternatives.

Here are 16 nourishments that might be deserving of the regarded super food title.

1. Dim Leafy Greens

Dim green verdant vegetables (DGLVs) are a magnificent wellspring of supplements including folate, zinc, calcium, iron, magnesium, nutrient C and fiber.

Some portion of what makes DGLVs so super is their capability to diminish your danger of ceaseless sicknesses including coronary illness and type 2 diabetes.

They likewise contain significant levels of mitigating mixes known as carotenoids, which may ensure against particular sorts of malignant growth.

Some notable DGLVs include:

Kale

Swiss chard

Collard greens

Turnip greens

Spinach

Some DGLVs have a harsh taste and not every person appreciates them plain. You can get imaginative by remembering them for your preferred soups, servings of mixed greens, smoothies, sautés and curries.

Synopsis

Dull green verdant vegetables are brimming with fiber and supplements which might be instrumental in forestalling certain incessant illnesses.

2. Berries

Berries are a healthful powerhouse of nutrients, minerals, fiber and cell reinforcements.

The solid cell reinforcement limit of berries is related with a diminished danger of coronary illness, malignant growth and other incendiary conditions.

Berries may likewise be successful in treating different stomach related and resistant related issue when utilized close by conventional medicinal treatments.

Probably the most widely recognized berries include:

Raspberries

Strawberries

Blueberries

Blackberries

Cranberries

Regardless of whether you appreciate them as a component of your morning meal, as a treat, on a plate of mixed greens or in a smoothie, the medical advantages of berries are as flexible as their culinary applications.

Outline

Berries are loaded with supplements and cell reinforcements which may forestall certain illnesses and improve absorption.

3. Green Tea

Initially from China, green tea is a delicately jazzed refreshment with a wide exhibit of restorative properties.

Green tea is wealthy in cancer prevention agents and polyphenolic mixes which have solid mitigating impacts. One of the most common cell reinforcements in green tea is the catechin epigallocatechin gallate, or EGCG.

EGCG is likely what gives green tea its clear capacity to ensure against ceaseless sicknesses including coronary illness, diabetes and disease.

Research likewise demonstrates that the blend of catechins and caffeine in green tea may make it a viable instrument for weight loss in certain individuals.

Rundown

Green tea is cell reinforcement rich with numerous medical advantages including conceivable malignant growth avoidance.

4. Eggs

Eggs have truly been a disputable point in the nourishment world because of their elevated cholesterol content, yet they stay perhaps the most advantageous nourishment.

Entire eggs are plentiful in numerous supplements including B nutrients, choline, selenium, nutrient An, iron and phosphorus.

They're additionally stacked with top notch protein.

Eggs contain two strong cancer prevention agents, zeaxanthin and lutein, which are known to ensure vision and eye wellbeing.

In spite of fears encompassing egg utilization and elevated cholesterol, investigate demonstrates no quantifiable increment in coronary illness or diabetes hazard from eating up to 6–12 eggs for each week.

Truth be told, eating eggs could expand "great" HDL cholesterol in certain individuals, which may prompt a good decrease in coronary illness hazard. More research is expected to reach a distinct determination.

Rundown

Eggs are wealthy in great protein and one of a kind cancer prevention agents. Research demonstrates that eating eggs normally won't expand your danger of coronary illness or diabetes.

5. Vegetables

Vegetables, or heartbeats, are a class of plant nourishments made up of beans (counting soy), lentils, peas, peanuts and horse feed.

They procure the super food mark since they're stacked with supplements and assume a job in forestalling and overseeing different maladies.

Vegetables are a rich wellspring of B nutrients, different minerals, protein and fiber.

Research shows that they offer numerous medical advantages including improved sort 2 diabetes the board, just as decreased circulatory strain and cholesterol.

Eating beans and vegetables routinely may likewise advance sound weight support, because of their capacity to improve sentiments of completion.

Outline

Vegetables are plentiful in numerous nutrients, protein and fiber. They may forestall some constant infections and bolster weight loss.

6. Nuts and Seeds

Nuts and seeds are wealthy in fiber, veggie lover protein and heart-solid fats.

They additionally pack different plant mixes with calming and cell reinforcement properties, which can secure against oxidative pressure.

Research shows that eating nuts and seeds can have a defensive impact against coronary illness.

Basic nuts and seeds include:

Almonds, walnuts, pistachios, pecans, cashews, Brazil nuts, macadamia nuts.

Peanuts — in fact a vegetable, yet often thought to be a nut.

Sunflower seeds, pumpkin seeds, chia seeds, flaxseeds, hemp seeds.

Strikingly, despite the fact that nuts and seeds are calorically thick, a few kinds of nuts are connected to weight loss when remembered for a decent diet.

Rundown

Nuts and seeds are brimming with fiber and heart-sound fats. They may lessen your danger of coronary illness and bolster weight loss.

7. Kefir (And Yogurt)

Kefir is a matured drink generally produced using milk that contains protein, calcium, B nutrients, potassium and probiotics.

Kefir is like yogurt yet has a more slender consistency and regularly more probiotic strains than yogurt.

Aged, probiotic-rich nourishments like kefir have a few related medical advantages, including decreased cholesterol, brought down pulse, improved absorption and calming impacts.

Despite the fact that kefir is generally produced using dairy animals' milk, it's ordinarily all around endured by individuals with lactose prejudice because of the maturation of the lactose by microscopic organisms.

Nonetheless, it's likewise produced using non-dairy drinks, for example, coconut milk, rice milk and coconut water.

You can buy kefir or make it yourself. If you're picking a financially arranged item, be aware of included sugar.

Outline

Kefir is an aged dairy drink with numerous medical advantages identified with its probiotic content. In spite of the fact that by and large produced using bovine's milk, kefir is additionally accessible in non-dairy structures.

8. Garlic

Garlic is a plant nourishment that is firmly identified with onions, leeks and shallots. It's a decent wellspring of manganese, nutrient C, nutrient B6, selenium and fiber.

Garlic is a mainstream culinary fixing because of its unmistakable flavor, however it has likewise been utilized for its therapeutic advantages for a considerable length of time.

Research shows that garlic might be powerful in diminishing cholesterol and circulatory strain, just as supporting invulnerable capacity.

In addition, sulfur-containing mixes in garlic may even assume a job in forestalling specific sorts of malignant growth.

Outline

Garlic is a supplement rich nourishment utilized for its restorative advantages for a considerable length of time. It might be helpful for supporting invulnerable capacity and lessening your danger of coronary illness and certain tumors.

9. Olive Oil

Olive oil is a characteristic oil extricated from the product of olive trees and one of the pillars of the Mediterranean diet.

It's greatest cases to wellbeing are its significant levels of monounsaturated unsaturated fats (MUFAs) and polyphenolic mixes.

Adding olive oil to your diet may diminish irritation and your danger of specific ailments, for example, coronary illness and diabetes.

It additionally contains cancer prevention agents, for example, nutrients E and K, which can shield against cell harm from oxidative pressure.

Outline

Olive oil is one of the standard fat sources in the Mediterranean diet. It might be valuable in lessening coronary illness, diabetes and other provocative conditions.

10. Ginger

Ginger originates from the foundation of a blossoming plant from China. It's utilized as both a culinary flavor enhancer and for its numerous restorative impacts.

Ginger root contains cell reinforcements, for example, gingerol, that might be answerable for huge numbers of the announced medical advantages related with this nourishment.

Ginger might be successful for overseeing queasiness and lessening torment from intense and constant fiery conditions.

It might likewise lessen your danger of constant sicknesses, for example, coronary illness, dementia and certain malignant growths.

Ginger is accessible crisp, as an oil or squeeze and in dried/powdered structures. It's anything but difficult to fuse into soups, sautés, sauces and teas.

Outline

Ginger is utilized for its flavor and potential restorative impacts. It might be valuable in treating sickness, torment and forestalling certain interminable illnesses.

11. Turmeric (Curcumin)

Turmeric is a brilliant yellow flavor that is firmly identified with ginger. Initially from India, it's utilized for cooking and its restorative advantages.

Curcumin is the dynamic compound in turmeric. It has intense cancer prevention agent and mitigating impacts and is the focal point of most research encompassing turmeric.

Studies show that curcumin might be powerful in treating and forestalling constant infections, for example, malignancy, coronary illness and diabetes.

It might likewise help wound mending and agony decrease.

One downside of utilizing curcumin restoratively is that it's not effectively consumed by your body, yet its ingestion can be improved by matching it with fats or different flavors, for example, dark pepper.

Outline

The dynamic compound in turmeric, curcumin, is related with a few restorative impacts. Curcumin isn't effectively retained and ought to be combined with substances that upgrade its assimilation, for example, dark pepper.

12. Salmon

Salmon is a profoundly nutritious fish stuffed with sound fats, protein, B nutrients, potassium and selenium.

It's probably the best wellspring of omega-3 unsaturated fats, which are known for an assortment of medical advantages, for example, diminishing irritation.

Remembering salmon for your diet may likewise bring down your danger of coronary illness and diabetes and assist you with keeping up a sound weight.

A potential disadvantage of eating salmon and different kinds of fish is their conceivable tainting with substantial metals and other natural poisons.

You can stay away from potential negative impacts by restricting your utilization of fish to a few servings for every week (41).

Synopsis

Salmon is a decent wellspring of numerous supplements, particularly omega-3 unsaturated fats. Point of confinement your utilization of salmon to keep away from potential negative impacts from contaminants basic in fish and fish.

13. Avocado

Avocado is an exceptionally nutritious natural product, however it's often treated progressively like a vegetable in culinary applications.

It's plentiful in numerous supplements, including fiber, nutrients, minerals and sound fats.

Like olive oil, avocado is high in monounsaturated fats (MUFAs). Oleic corrosive is the most transcendent MUFA in avocado, which is connected to diminished irritation in the body.

Eating avocado may decrease your danger of coronary illness, diabetes, metabolic disorder and specific kinds of malignant growth.

Outline

Avocados are supplement rich, high-fiber natural products that may assume a job in diminishing irritation and ceaseless infections.

14. Sweet Potato

The sweet potato is a root vegetable stacked with numerous supplements, including potassium, fiber and nutrients An and C.

They're additionally a decent wellspring of carotenoids, a sort of cell reinforcement that may lessen your danger of specific kinds of malignant growth.

In spite of their sweet flavor, sweet potatoes don't build glucose as much as you would anticipate. Curiously, they may really improve glucose control in those with type 2 diabetes.

Outline

Sweet potatoes are a profoundly nutritious nourishment stacked with carotenoids, which have solid cell reinforcement properties. They may likewise be advantageous for glucose control.

15. Mushrooms

The absolute most regular assortments of eatable mushrooms are button, portobello, shiitake, crimini and clam mushrooms.

Despite the fact that supplement content changes relying upon the sort, mushrooms contain nutrient A, potassium, fiber, and a few cell reinforcements not present in most different nourishments.

Strikingly, eating more mushrooms is related with more noteworthy utilization of vegetables all in all, adding to a general progressively nutritious diet.

Because of their one of a kind cell reinforcement content, mushrooms may likewise assume a job in lessening irritation and forestalling specific sorts of malignancies.

Another super element of mushrooms is that rural waste items are utilized to develop them. This makes mushrooms a supportable part of a sound nourishment framework.

Outline

Mushrooms are loaded with supplements and may decrease your danger of specific ailments. Furthermore, mushrooms are a manageable nourishment decision.

16. Kelp

Kelp is a term used to portray certain supplement rich ocean vegetables. It's most normally devoured in Asian food however is picking up notoriety in different pieces of the world because of its healthy benefit.

Ocean growth packs numerous supplements, including nutrient K, folate, iodine and fiber.

These sea vegetables are a wellspring of novel bioactive mixes — not ordinarily show in land-vegetables — which may have cell reinforcement impacts.

A portion of these mixes may likewise diminish your danger of malignant growth, coronary illness, heftiness and diabetes.

Synopsis

Ocean growth is a gathering of exceptionally nutritious ocean vegetables that may assume a job in ensuring against certain interminable illnesses.

1. Greek Yogurt Regular yogurt's thicker, creamier cousin is crammed with protein and probiotics. It fills the gut, improves absorption, and reinforces the insusceptible framework. Furthermore, it's an extraordinary sound formula substitute for sharp cream, cream cheddar, and even mayonnaise!

2. Quinoa This minuscule, grain-like seed packs some genuine dietary ability. With a mellow, nutty flavor and a surface like rice or couscous, quinoa is one of the main grains or seeds that gives every one of the nine basic amino acids our bodies can't deliver themselves. Also, it's loaded up with protein—eight grams for each one-cup serving, to be careful!

3. Blueberries Don't stress; these berries won't cause an oompa-loompa-like response. Actually, they're wholesome geniuses, loaded up with fiber, nutrient C, and malignancy battling mixes. Furthermore, considers propose blueberries may even improve memory!

4. Kale This unpleasant and intense green prevails over all the rest regarding sustenance, giving a greater number of cancer prevention agents than most different foods grown from the ground! It's likewise a phenomenal wellspring of fiber, calcium, and iron. Set it

up basically any way, from bubbled or steamed to broiled (attempt it as a chip!) or stewed.

5. Chia Ch-ch-ch-chia! That's right, this little seed is equivalent to those delightful minimal artistic creature grower of the 90s! In any case, don't stress, the nutritious part isn't the dirt pot. Chia seeds are really stacked with the most basic unsaturated fats of any known plant! Additionally, one serving of the stuff is stacked with magnesium, iron, calcium, and potassium.

6. Cereal High in fiber, cell reinforcements, and huge amounts of different supplements, this morning meal staple has been appeared to help lower cholesterol levels, help in processing, and even improve digestion. What's more, it's out and out scrumptious—particularly when seasoned like pumpkin pie!

7. Green Tea This ages-old wellbeing mystery has been utilized as a characteristic solution for everything from malignant growth to coronary illness! The key to this heavenly drink? Cell reinforcements! The fundamental hero here is Epigallocatechin gallate, or EGCG, a phytochemical that eases back unpredictable cell development, which might help forestall the development of certain malignancies.

8. Broccoli This lean, mean, green machine is pressed with nutrients, minerals, ailment battling mixes, and the fiber basic in any diet. In spite of the fact that all individuals from the cruciferous vegetable family are super sound, broccoli stands apart for its outstandingly elevated levels of nutrient C and folate (which can diminish danger of coronary illness, certain tumors, and stroke).

9.Strawberries Vitamin C is the genius of this super food. Only one cup of these red wonders fulfills the everyday necessity for nutrient C (74 milligrams for each day for ladies, 90 for men)! Studies propose the cell reinforcement helps fabricate and fix the body's tissues, supports insusceptibility, and battles overabundance free extreme harm. What's more, the nutrient C in strawberries could help advance solid eye work.

10. Salmon This heart-solid fish is pressed with protein and a sound portion of omega-3 unsaturated fats, which studies recommend may help diminish the danger of cardiovascular illness. What's more, extra focuses: Salmon may likewise shield skin from the sun and the harming impacts of UV beams.

11. Watermelon Low in sugar and high in nutrients An and C, this midyear treat is the ideal, amazing failure calorie nibble. Studies recommend watermelon could likewise possibly bring down circulatory strain and diminish the danger of cardiovascular sickness. Furthermore, the lycopene in watermelon could help shield the body from UV beams and malignant growth.

12. Spinach Antioxidants, hostile to inflammatory, and nutrients that advance vision and bone wellbeing are what make this green so super. What's more, those bones will thank spinach, as well! Only one cup of the stuff gets together to 12 percent of the suggested day by day portion of calcium and enough nutrient K to help forestall bone loss.

13. Pistachios These lil' nuts are concealing loads of protein and fiber behind their hearty flavor and nutty crunch. In addition, they're normally sans cholesterol. A one-ounce serving of these nuts has nearly as a lot of potassium as one little banana.

14. Eggs A moderately cheap protein source stacked with supplements, eggs positively acquire their super food status. A solitary huge egg is just around 70 calories and offers six grams of protein. Eggs are

likewise an extraordinary wellspring of omega-3 unsaturated fats, which are fundamental for ordinary body capacity and heart wellbeing.

15. Almonds Surprise! Almonds are the most healthfully thick nut, which means they offer the most elevated centralization of supplements per calorie per ounce. For only 191 calories, a one-ounce serving gives 3.4 grams of fiber (that is around 14 percent of the everyday suggested esteem) and a solid portion of potassium, calcium, nutrient E, magnesium, and iron. Furthermore, you can eat them as BUTTER!

16. Ginger Slightly zesty yet quite pleasant, ginger has been utilized for quite a long time as a delectable enhancing and an all-characteristic solution for everything from a steamed stomach to undesirable irritation.

17. Beets This elite player veggie contains huge amounts of nutrients, minerals, and cell reinforcements that can help battle ailment and strengthen indispensable organs. Also, their purple tint might be the key to their sound achievement—a few examinations recommend betalains, the purple shades

in these veggies, may assist ward with offing malignant growth and other degenerative sicknesses.

18. Beans High in protein and low in cholesterol, beans of any assortment can add a sound wind to any dish (even brownies!). They're likewise stacked with fiber, folate, and magnesium, and studies have demonstrated that vegetables (like beans) can really help lower cholesterol and decrease the danger of specific diseases (at any rate in rodents...).

19. Pumpkin Loaded with cancer prevention agents and nutrients, these gourds aren't only for cutting (or making into pie). The star supplement here is beta-carotene, a provitamin that the body changes over to nutrient A, which is known for its resistant boosting forces and fundamental job in eye wellbeing.

20. Apples Say it with us, individuals: "Fiber is acceptable." And apples are an incredible low-calorie source. (A medium-sized apple tips the scales at under 100 calories.) Plus, increasing apple consumption has been related with decreased danger of cardiovascular sickness, certain malignant growths, diabetes, and asthma.

21. Cranberries It's an ideal opportunity to work these fall top choices into dishes all year. Regardless of whether it's looking like a can or new off the stove, cranberries have a bunch of medical advantages and illness battling powers. These microscopic organisms busting berries can help battle irritation, lessen the danger of coronary illness, improve oral wellbeing, help forestall ulcers and yeast contaminations, and may even restrain the development of some human malignant growth cells.

22. Garlic Yes, it may leave breath not exactly attractive, yet these cloves can accomplish more than season—they've been utilized for a considerable length of time as nourishment and drug. Nowadays, garlic is utilized to treat anything from hypertension and coronary illness to specific kinds of malignant growth. Also, considers recommend garlic concentrate can be utilized to treat yeast diseases in ladies and prostate issues in men.

23. Cauliflower While every one of the nutrients and minerals are an extraordinary reward, the genuine star here is cauliflower's disease battling mixes, glucosinolates. These phytochemicals are answerable

for cauliflower's occasionally harsh flavor, yet they have additionally been appeared to forestall harm to the lungs and stomach via cancer-causing agents, possibly ensuring against those malignant growths. Furthermore, on account of communications with estrogen, cauliflower may likewise help forestall hormone-driven malignant growths like bosom, uterine, and cervical.

SIRTFOOD RECIPE

Super foods are probably the most healthfully thick nourishments on earth. While a considerable lot of us are simply getting on to the super food pattern, many have been utilized for a huge number of years by indigenous individuals as different types of common prescription. These force stuffed nourishments arrive in an assortment of structures from seeds, berries, gels and powders, each accompanying a different advantage.

1. Orange, Fig and Baobab Cheesecake

Recall the baobab tree from "The Little Prince?" Who might have believed that baobab was a super food in addition to it tastes extraordinary! This Orange, Fig and Baobab Cheesecake is a tasty, velvety treat that is made altogether of common entire nourishments so you can appreciate each significant piece!

2. Goji Berry and Hazelnut Cacao Truffles

Goji berries are little yet enthusiastic about nourishment. These Goji Berry and Hazelnut Cacao Truffles are abounded in squashed goji berries. They're brisk and simple, crude, veggie lover, sans gluten, without dairy, paleo-accommodating, no-heat, and no have no refined sugar. Gracious definitely, they're extremely scrumptious as well!

3. Mint Matcha Chip Ice Cream

This Mint Matcha Chocolate Chip Ice Cream is smooth, liberal and bravo! It has matcha green tea in it which gives it shading as well as it's a super food. In addition to the fact that this is anything but difficult to make thus reviving, it'll immediately turn into your new most loved flavor!

4. Bubbly Coconut, Lime and Mint Kombucha Elixir

This Fizzy Coconut, Lime and Mint Kombucha Elixir is reviving, tastes astonishing, looks beautiful, is hydrating, feeding and loaded with solid probiotics! Both coconut and fermented tea are considered superfoods. Check out it at home and intrigue companions with this pretty mocktail.

5. Crude Chocolate Mint Grasshopper Pie

This Raw Chocolate Mint Grasshopper Pie is a genuine group pleaser and ideal for an uncommon event with loved ones. Where's the super food? Spirulina, a sort of green growth, gives this pie its beautiful shading and huge amounts of solid supplements.

6. Rainbow Vegetable Saffron Millet Croquettes

Antiquated grains are superfoods and it's enjoyable to attempt new ones you may not be comfortable with like millet. These Rainbow Vegetable Saffron Millet Croquettes are an incredible method to attempt it. The outside gets fresh and within remains delicate. You'll begin to look all starry eyed at this grain and this dish.

7. Kimchi Kale Salad

Aged nourishments are superfoods and an extraordinary method to get probiotics into your diet. Eating kimchi, a Korean dish like sauerkraut, is a heavenly method to do it. Kimchi includes such a lot of flavor, surface, and shading to nourishment. The crunch and harshness are particularly brilliant right now Salad made with avocado, kneaded kale, chickpeas, and broiled sweet potatoes – which all happen to be superfoods too.

8. Hand crafted Dark Chocolate Chunks

Genuine chocolate – the sort accepted to hold enchanted, or even celestial, properties. All things considered, we have been hearing that a tad of dim chocolate is useful for the heart and certainly for the spirit. This Homemade Dark Chocolate Chunks formula lets you control the measure of sweetness and salt in your chocolate. That is the excellence of making your own.

9. Broiled Cauliflower and Avocado Cream Pitas

Cauliflower and avocado are both dietary powerhouses and these Roasted Cauliflower and Avocado Cream Pitas are the most tasty approach to practice good eating habits. The spiced broiled cauliflower and avocado cream are an agreeable flavor blend that preferences great on totally anything.

10. Best Ever Forbidden Rice Salad

Dark rice is a super food and the way that it's called prohibited rice just makes it much progressively captivating. This Forbidden Rice Salad is simple, fast, and ensured to intrigue. Dark rice has a simmered nutty flavor and matches well with a wide range of veggies and greens. The ginger miso dressing goes splendidly with the sweet potatoes and nutty rice.

11. Zesty Kale and Quinoa Black Bean Salad

Kale and quinoa are both superfoods. When you set up them with solid dark beans right now and Quinoa Black Bean Salad, you have a wholesome trifecta! Dark colored rice, dark beans, peppers, corn, salsa, lettuce, guacamole – what's not to adore?

12. Chia Pudding With Blueberries

Chia seeds are sound and berries are additionally superfoods. This Chia Pudding with Blueberries is smooth, sweet and sustaining. This treat is so liberal and delectable, you'll overlook it's beneficial for you.

13. Plantain Sweet Potato Tacos With Guacamole

These Plantain Sweet Potato Tacos with Guacamole are actually as they sound – loaded down with plantains, sweet potatoes and dark beans and bested with a basic guacamole. They're veggie lover, sans gluten and a phenomenal lunch or supper alternative!

14. Chocolate Einkorn Cake

Is it cake? Is it a brownie? Whatever you call it, this Chocolate Einkorn Cake is delightful. It's a super chocolately, not excessively sweet, wet cake-brownie bar ... and it's incredible. Einkorn wheat is old wheat that has never been hereditarily modified so it's solid and simpler to process.

15. Coconut Flour Porridge With Roasted Apricots

Did you realize that coconut flour makes a thick and delightful gluten and without grain porridge? Disregard your common cereal and attempt this yummy, simple breakfast of Coconut Flour Porridge! It's particularly delicious when topped with sweet caramelized apricots, however mess around with your own preferred garnishes.

16. Sound Hearty Whole Wheat Pancakes With Flax

It's constantly enjoyable to add foods grown from the ground to the hitter yet in some cases you need a flapjack formula that is somewhat more unbiased in enhance. A formula that asks for sweet fixings and a streaming waterway of maple syrup. However, obviously, it despite everything must be sound. These Healthy Hearty Whole Wheat Pancakes fit the bill impeccably. They top you off with Omega rich flax all while as yet tasting flavorful close by some new leafy foods mug of espresso or tea.

17. Spring Onion Farro Fritters With Fresh Peas, Asparagus, Radish and Tahini Mint Dressing

If farro is another grain for you, these Spring Onion Farro Fritters with Fresh Peas, Asparagus and Radishes are an extraordinary method to get presented. They are entire nourishments, plant-based thus scrumptious. Present with the mint tahini dressing which is tasty and furthermore solid.

18. Bahn Mi Salad With Pickled Vegetables and Vietnamese Croutons

Cured nourishments are superfoods and this Banh Mi Salad with Pickled Vegetables is a super dish. It's loaded up with dynamic flavors and the Vietnamese bread garnishes on top include crunch. This formula serves two huge plates of mixed greens and is veggie lover, protein-pressed and without nut with a sans gluten alternative accessible.

19. Crude Apple Pie With Goji Berries and Nutmeg

You might be thinking about how crusty fruit-filled treat can be a super food? When it's this Raw Apple Pie with Goji Berries and Nutmeg, it can. It has sound apples, super food goji berries and it's crude so there's no batter. It is as nutritious as it is delectable! It is additionally exquisite topped with coconut yogurt.

20. Avocado and Veggie Spring Rolls

Avocados are superfoods and we are so cheerful about that. These Avocado and Veggie Spring Rolls are so flavorful. Loaded up with crunchy veggies and velvety avocado with bunches of Asian flavors, we prescribe making a great deal in light of the fact that these will vanish before your eyes.

21. Broccoli and Coconut Soup

This Broccoli and Coconut Soup is a lively, delightful and exceptionally nutritious mix of broccoli, spinach, lemon, ginger, and coconut milk that will warm you and feed you through the cooler winter months or just whenever you have to heat up inside.

22. Wild Rice Salad With Orange, Sweet Potato, Cherries and Pecans

This Wild Rice Salad is so pretty thus bravo. It's overflowing with a wide range of superfoods. Zest up your typical plate of mixed greens life with this delicious mix of wild rice, sweet potato, orange, fruits, and walnuts. It's the best of fall in a bowl!

23. Dark Bean Hemp Burgers

These Black Bean Hemp Burgers are so ideal for lunch, supper, nibble, even breakfast. They're likewise an ideal travel partner that will get together effectively and keep you full for a considerable length of time, on account of all the protein, fiber, and supplements.

24. Fig Hazelnut Rosemary Granola With Fig Breakfast 'Decent' Cream

Dried figs are superfoods and they're doubly solid right now Rosemary Granola with Fig Breakfast 'Decent' Cream since they are utilized twice! This yummy breakfast combo has dried figs that make the granola magnificently chewy and solidified green figs zoomed up until cushy in the "pleasant" cream.

25. Green Bean and Wild Rice Salad

When served warm, this Green Bean and Wild Rice Salad is sufficiently healthy to eat during even the coldest winter months and it has a few superfoods in it. Crunchy almonds, chewy cranberries and sun-dried tomatoes, tart olives, and generous wild rice give an intriguing blend of surfaces that will make them desire more!

SCIENCE BEHIND SIRTFOODS

Hardly any things are so profoundly contaminated by trends, cheats and misrepresentation as nourishment. All things considered, it is through a perspective of sound wariness that we should see any new diet. The most recent to stand out as truly newsworthy is the Sirtfood diet which, if we are to fully trust claims, will help with weight loss just as offering different advantages, for example, "invigorating restoration and cell fix".

For the unenlightened, this most recent diet is based around utilization of nourishments which may associate with a group of proteins known as sirtuin proteins, or SIRT1 - SIRT7. Adding to the diet's undoubted request is the way that the best sources as far as anyone knows incorporate red wine and chocolate, just as citrus organic products, blueberries and kale. During the initial three days, calorie admission is restricted (1,000 calories for every day) and comprises of three Sirtfood green juices, in addition to a typical feast rich in "Sirtfoods". On days four to seven, calorie admission is expanded (1,500 calories) and comprises of two juices and two dinners. Past that the suggestion is to eat a reasonable diet rich in sirtuin nourishments, alongside further green juices. Prawns and salmon additionally include in the supper plans.

It sounds scrumptious – and sirtuins are for sure embroiled in a wide scope of cell forms including digestion, maturing and circadian musicality. The diet is additionally situated to a limited extent, on calorie limitation. The nutritionists behind this recommend the diet "impacts the body's capacity to consume fat and lifts the metabolic framework".

The diet decoded

So what do we think about this diet? From a scientific viewpoint, the appropriate response is: practically nothing. Sirtuins add to guideline of fat and glucose digestion in light of changes in vitality levels. They may likewise have an impact in the impact of calorie limitation on upgrades in maturing. This is maybe by means of sirtuins' consequences for high-impact (or mitochondrial) digestion, bringing down of responsive oxygen species (free radicals) and increments in cancer prevention agent proteins.

Besides, explore recommends that transgenic mice with more elevated levels of SIRT6 live significantly longer than wild-type mice, and that changes in SIRT6 articulation might be important in maturing of some human skin cells. SIRT2 likewise has been shownto moderate metazoan (yeast) maturing.

It sounds noteworthy and the diet makes them gleam surveys, however none of this speaks to convincing scientific proof of the Sirtfood Diet effect sly affecting genuine individuals. It would be a colossal over-extrapolation to expect that lab look into directed on mice, yeast and human undifferentiated organisms has any bearing on certifiable wellbeing results – polluted as they are by a huge number of perplexing factors.

The study of weight loss

Surely the diet will seem to work for certain individuals. Be that as it may, scientific evidence of any diet's triumphs is an altogether different issue. Obviously, the perfect investigation to think about the adequacy of a diet on weight loss (or some other result, for example, maturing) would require an adequately huge example – agent of the populace we are keen on – and arbitrary allotment to a treatment or control gathering. Results would then be checked over a satisfactory timeframe with severe command over perplexing factors, for example, different practices that may emphatically or contrarily influence the results of enthusiasm (smoking, for example, or work out).

This exploration would be constrained by techniques, for example, self-detailing and memory, yet would go some approach to finding the viability of this diet. Research of this nature, be that as it may, doesn't exist and we ought to therefore be careful when deciphering fundamental science – all things considered, human cells in a tissue culture dish likely respond differently to the phones in a living individual.

Further uncertainty is thrown over this diet when we think about a portion of the specific cases. Losses of seven pounds in a single week are unreasonable and are probably not going to reflect changes to muscle versus fat. For the initial three days, dieters expend around 1000 kcal every day – around 40–half of what the vast majority require. This will bring about a quick loss of glycogen (a put away type of sugar) from skeletal muscle and the liver.

In any case, for each gram of put away glycogen we likewise store around 2.7 grams of water, and water is overwhelming. So for all the lost glycogen, we additionally lose going with water – and thus weight. Also, diets that are too prohibitive are extremely difficult to follow and bring about increments in hunger invigorating hormones, for example, ghrelin. Weight (glycogen and water) will therefore come back to ordinary if the desire to eat wins out.

When all is said in done, utilization of the scientific strategy to the investigation of nourishment is difficult. It is often impractical to complete fake treatment controlled preliminaries with any level of natural legitimacy, and the wellbeing results that we are often keen on happen over numerous years, making research configuration testing. Besides, contemplates in enormous populaces rely upon shockingly shortsighted and innocent information assortment techniques, for example, memory and self-detailing, which produce famously questionable information. Against this foundation commotion, nourishment look into has a difficult activity.

Is there a convenient solution?

Sadly, not. Sensationalized features and often hyperbolic portrayal of scientific information brings about the apparently unlimited contentions about what – and how much – we ought to eat, further fuelling our fixation on a "handy solution" or wonder fix, which in itself is an endemic social issue.

For the reasons sketched out, the Sirtfood diet ought to be relegated to the prevailing fashion heap – in any event from a scientific point of view. In light of the proof we have, to propose in any case is, best case scenario false and even under the least favorable conditions deluding and harming to the real points of general wellbeing procedure. The diet is probably not going to offer any profit to populaces confronting a plague of diabetes, prowling in the shadow of weight. As expressed obviously by others, exceptional diets don't work and dieting all in all is anything but a general wellbeing answer for social orders where the greater part of grown-ups are overweight.

By and by, the best system is long haul conduct change joined with political and ecological impact, focused on expanded physical movement and some type of cognizant authority over what we eat. It is anything but a convenient solution, yet it will work.

There's another big name diet on the square, and it's sponsored by none other than Adele. The British vocalist lyricist's emotional change and right around 50-pound weight loss got everybody discussing the Sirtfood Diet – which includes initiating your 'thin quality' by remembering certain nourishments for your diet. Chocolate, red wine and espresso are not beyond reach and you can lose as much as seven pounds every week.

Like most prevailing fashion diets, it sounds excessively great to be valid, or possibly, feasible. In this way, here's a more intensive look.

What goes into it?

The term 'sirt nourishments' was promoted not long ago by British nutritionists Aidan Goggins and Glen Matten with the arrival of their book, The Sirtfood Diet. It advocates a diet wealthy in nourishments that invigorate sirtuin, a specific protein accepted to advance weight loss through accelerating digestion and expanding strong proficiency. Sirtuins are additionally connected with life span since it forestalls aggravation and advances cell development.

The diet itself is comprised of two phases. During the initial three days of stage one, calorie admission is restricted to 1000 cals a day spread across three sirtfood green juices and one standard feast with sirtuin-rich nourishments. In days 4–7, 1500 calories are devoured through two juices and two standard suppers daily. In arrange two, which endures 14 days, dieters eat three adjusted sirtfood-rich suppers alongside one serving of green juice. Post that, the proposal is to eat a fair diet rich in sirtuin nourishments and green juices. The creators demand that the Sirtfood Diet centers on eating the nourishments you love and not removing food sources or slandering entire nutritional categories.

Sirtuin-rich nourishments

Fortunately the sirtuin-rich nourishments suggested by the book are all around nutritious and useful for a great many people. These incorporate pecans, strawberries, espresso, kale, celery with leaves, additional virgin olive oil, buckwheat, stew, cocoa (in any event 85-percent unadulterated), matcha, green tea, medjool dates, red chicory, red onion, red wine, arugula, soy and turmeric.

The green juice contains Kale, parsley, rocket, celery, apple, lemon and matcha.

GREENS

Does it work?

Any diet that confines your calorie-admission is probably going to work at the outset and individuals have detailed dropping numbers on the scale. Be that as it may, is this weight loss practical? "Regarding weight loss and boosting digestion, individuals may have encountered a seven pound weight loss on the scales, yet as far as I can tell this will be liquid. Consuming and losing fat requires significant investment so it is amazingly far-fetched this weight loss is a loss of fat," dietitian Emer Delaney clarifies in BBC Good Food.

The genuine test lies in guaranteeing that the weight remains off and your body gets all its basic supplements simultaneously. While there's no denying that the sirtfoods prescribed are in fact sound, there's constantly a peril of overabundance. A lot of cocoa, wine or olive oil will include calories regardless. Also, calorie necessities rely upon your tallness, sexual orientation and action levels, so there's actually nobody size-fit-all diet

Discontinuous fasting (IF) has huge amounts of advantages, including weight loss, forestalling diabetes, and lessening your danger of disease. Numerous individuals who follow IF state that it's helped them appreciate their dinners more and comprehend the difference among appetite and desires. It has likewise helped them get through weight loss levels.

"IF causes you to feel great since you're disposing of the aggravation," says, Wendy Scinta, M.D., leader of the Obesity Medicine Association and an individual from Prevention's Medical Review Board. "I follow the 16:8 diet and find that when I endorse IF to patients who need to shed 100 pounds and can't lose the last 15 pounds, IF causes them arrive."

In any case, IF isn't for everybody (Dr. Scinta doesn't suggest it for individuals who have a background marked by scattered eating or pregnant ladies), and it's essential to comprehend the symptoms that accompany it.

Regardless of what sort of irregular fasting technique you're keen on following, here are symptoms you should know.

1. Beginners may feel hypoglycemic.

From the outset, you may encounter hypoglycemia, a condition brought about by extremely low glucose levels. This can prompt migraines, expanded pulse, dazedness, and queasiness, according to Dr. Scinta. Goodness, and awful dispositions—nobody's cheerful when they're confining nourishment. "When you don't eat, your body will initially consume the glycogen (put away glucose) in your liver and muscles (subsequently feeling aggravated from the start), then it will start to consume fat for fuel," says Frances Largeman-Roth, R.D.N., nourishment and wellbeing master, creator of Eating in Color and maker of the FLR VIP program, says. In any case, as your body turns out to be more keto versatile and figures out how to run on fat rather than glucose, Dr. Scinta says hypoglycemia turns out to be to a lesser extent a worry.

In any case, if you keep on feeling woozy or bleary eyed after some time, Largeman-Roth says to eat something—regardless of whether it's a little bite.

"Shedding pounds is never an adequate motivation to drop," she says.

What's more, make a point to fuel up on solid, fulfilling nourishments during suppers. Slender protein, leafy foods, entire grains, and sound fats, for example, avocados, nuts, and extra-virgin olive oil will keep your glucose levels adjusted during your quick and give the supplements your body needs to work appropriately.

Dr. Scinta says she often finds that individuals on IF battle to get enough protein, so make sure to eat routinely, including tidbits, when you're not fasting. "You should plan to get at any rate one gram of protein for each kilogram of weight every day," she says.

2. You'll hunger for carbs and prepared nourishments less.

Dr. Scinta says that numerous individuals who follow IF make some better memories at keeping their glucose levels adjusted. In such a case that powers you to quit eating at a specific time, you'll fuel up on all the more fulfilling nourishments, similar to lean protein and fiber, to remain full during your quick. "What I've found with IF is that it's helped me watch my carb consumption," Dr. Scinta says. "You're eating to such an extent, however you're not eating as a significant part of the terrible stuff."

IF additionally advances satiety through the creation of craving decreasing hormones. A recent report from Obesity recommends that IF can help decline ghrelin levels—the hormone that animates hunger—in overweight grown-ups and improve individuals' capacity to switch between consuming carbs for vitality and consuming fat for vitality.

"There are people who eat around evening time because of fatigue or stress, not on the grounds that they're really ravenous. Putting guardrails on the occasions they can eat may assist them with abstaining from eating when they don't should be," Largeman-Roth says.

Dr. Scinta and Largeman-Roth additionally encourage individuals to remain hydrated while fasting since individuals will in general mistake hunger for hunger.

"When individuals quick in the first part of the day, they drink a great deal of espresso, which is a diuretic, and neglect to drink water," Dr. Scinta says. "Each capacity in the body requires water, so remaining hydrated is unfathomably significant," Largeman-Roth says. "We get about 20% of our water consumption from the nourishment we eat, so when we quick, we're losing a significant wellspring of hydration," she says.

3. You'll improve your insulin affectability.

A recent report in Cell Metabolism found that men with pre-diabetes who followed IF improved their insulin affectability, despite the fact that they didn't get thinner. How can it work, precisely? Whenever you eat, your body discharges the hormone insulin to move sugar from your circulatory system into your cells for vitality. Be that as it may, individuals with pre-diabetes don't react well to insulin so their glucose levels remain raised. Expanding the time between suppers can help on the grounds that your body discharges less insulin.

In any case, Dr. Scinta says that individuals who are on insulin-subordinate drugs ought to counsel with their primary care physician before following IF in light of the fact that it can influence the adequacy of their treatment. "Individuals with type 1 or 2 diabetes are on these meds to bring down their glucose, so they have to have steady dinners to forestall spikes in their glucose," Dr. Scinta says.

4. Your workouts may endure a shot.

Following IF and working out is absolutely protected, however you'll have to make a few acclimations to your timetable with the goal that you're not running on void. Let's assume you're following the 5:2 diet: Doing low-affect workouts rather than progressively serious ones, similar to weight lifting, running, and HIIT, on days when you're constraining calories can enable your body to change in accordance with the new requests. As your body becomes acclimated to consuming fat for fuel, the power of your workouts won't be as a lot of a worry.

So, the exact opposite thing you need to do is drop during your HIIT class, so Dr. Scinta prescribes timing your workouts toward the start or end of your quick. Along these lines, you can appreciate a pre-or post-workout nibble. Nourishments that are anything but difficult to process, similar to a smoothie, low-fat yogurt, and nutty spread with toast work better pre-workout, while nourishments with a higher carb-to-protein proportion, for example, a bowl of cereal, are perfect for post-workout.

Researchers drove by Dr Naiara Beraza at the Institute of Food Research on the Norwich Research Park are exploring the systems supporting the alleged useful impacts of the 'Sirtfood Diet'.

Sirtfoods burst onto the wellbeing and sustenance scene prior this year, making a sprinkle in the media, with a few prominent competitors including Olympic gold-medallist Sir Ben Ainslie changing over their dietary propensities according to The Independent.

While this news may urge potential dieters to head out close by such brandishing VIPs, analysts at the IFR are provisional and propose unquestionably more research is required into the scientific premise behind the physiological advantages that the nourishments included are intended to convey.

So what is the scientific proof behind these cases?

A large number of these nourishments may to be sure have medical advantages for us when we eat them. There is acceptable proof that individuals who have diets high in vegetables and organic products have a decreased danger of creating ceaseless conditions. A portion of these nourishments contain bioactives, which are natural particles that impact living cells, and that may likewise show medical advantages. IFR has a program of research taking a gander at bioactives, to attempt to locate the best proof for how they are processed and the components by which they may profit wellbeing.

There are a wide range of manners by which these advantages might be deciphered. Defenders of the SIRTFOOD diet guarantee that bioactive mixes initiate proteins called sirtuins. These sirtuins trigger the statement of qualities that they connect to cell restoration and fix, concealment of craving and weight loss. Nourishments rich in these bioactives have been marked 'sirtfoods'; predominantly products of the soil including blueberries, rocket, celery, kale and apples and other nourishment types, for example, 85% dim chocolate and red wine. In any case, the proof connecting these sirtfoods back to human medical advantages, by means of enactment of sirtuins, is as yet uncertain.

We realize that there are seven sirtuins in our body yet we don't have the foggiest idea what they all do. The most notable is sirtuin 1. There is proof from tests in mice that overexpressing SIRT1 gives sound maturing and that these mice are ensured against high fat diet-actuated metabolic disorder, described by corpulence and greasy liver. Resveratrol, a proposed SIRT bioactive found in the skin of red grapes, has been appeared to actuate the SIRT1 quality, dragging out the lifespan of lower living beings yet not warm blooded creatures. Flavonoids found in chocolate are likewise known to initiate SIRT1 in worms.

Dr Beraza proposes that the scientific premise utilized for advancement of this diet is doubtlessly founded on the effect of resveratrol expanding the lifespan of lower creatures, for example, sprouting yeast. The cell components by which resveratrol acts stay dubious and presently the medical advantages in people can't seem to be demonstrated indisputably.

Another significant point is that the measure of bioactive found in these nourishments might be not even close to enough to have any advantageous impacts. While it's demonstrated that certain bioactives can actuate SIRT1, we don't know whether the levels in nourishments in amounts that individuals normally eat can encourage this enactment. Different components to consider are that eating these nourishments may infer a decrease in calorie admission, as the greater part of the related nourishments will in general be lower in sugars and fats, with diminished calorie utilization known to actuate SIRT1. Exercise may likewise be expanded in people participating in such a diet as most diets prescribe expanded exercise. Exercise is known to incite SIRT1 action so the nourishment itself may not assume such a significant job.

So what move would it be advisable for us to make to additionally examine SIRT1?

Dr. Bereza proposes that we should attempt to characterize the instruments basic any helpful impacts and how SIRT1 overexpression ensures against a high fat diet. There might be specific conditions where a lot of SIRT1 movement could prompt unintended impacts. Late research indicated that SIRT1 overexpression in mice delivered hindered liver recovery and a few different papers by different research bunches have demonstrated that SIRT1 is exceptionally communicated in liver tumor tests... Sirtuin 1 is an amazing particle that controls basic metabolic pathways, cell assurance frameworks and manages provocative reaction so it is important to characterize in which organs SIRT1 has impacts, and what those impacts are.

While some work has been done on the liver with respect to these systems, there is a nonattendance of research which endeavors to characterize the job of SIRT1 in the liver-gut hub. Her group at the IFR will examine this job to show whether SIRT1 actuation must be organ specific to harvest the advantageous impacts with the goal that we may reason the best technique to deliver viable SIRT1-based medications.

So should perusers forsake the SIRT send?

"I think not" affirms Dr. Beraza "However simply because huge numbers of the 'Sirtfoods' can be incorporated as a major aspect of a sound lifestyle which is known to present other dietary advantages. Dieters would likewise be better encouraged to consolidate these nourishments, as a blend of the mixes will probably have more prominent favorable circumstances than eating one nourishment type alone. Pathways other than SIRT1 can be actuated, upgrading the helpful impacts while likewise making dinners less exhausting! It is additionally essential to join these nourishments with non-SIRT nourishments as a feature of a fair diet including protein and suggested levels of fat nearby customary exercise."

In general, the SIRT1 message is idealistic with regards to stoutness, high fat diets and metabolic disorder, yet so as to expand the potential that these bioactives may have, we should completely examine the instruments behind these impacts, with specific accentuation on the job of SIRT in the liver-gut pivot. While an 'enchantment pill' to fix weight may at present be distant, work at the IFR could reveal more insight into the mind boggling systems embroiled in SIRT1 articulation to all the more likely comprehend a conceivably helpful dietary road.

CONCLUSION

'We don't yet have the proof that specific nourishments actuate this more than others – or to which specific tissues they'd be gainful,' says Hirschey. 'Regardless of whether sirtfoods do trigger weight loss, the sheer amount we'd have to eat might be unmanageable.' He focuses to resveratrol, the polyphenol in red wine and the most notable of all sirtuin activators.

Resveratrol shot to popularity in 2003 when a research facility run by David Sinclair found that this compound, found most normally in the skins of red grapes, copied the impacts of calorie limitation and actuated sirtuins that drawn out the life of cells. Subsequently the 'red wine encourages you live more' way of thinking that is become progressively mainstream bandied about at the bar.

Be that as it may, Hirschey brings up, 'most of studies have been done utilizing test frameworks in the lab, generally on mice or natural product flies, or legitimately into cells. To get resveratrol's enemy of maturing impacts from red wine, you'd need to drink up to 40 liters every day.' This makes you wonder how much kale you should pack so as to get thinner.

The nutraceutical business is as of now one stage ahead, with resveratrol supplements effectively accessible. Be watchful, in any case, of simply popping some sirt-enacting pills or binding your smoothies with resveratrol powder, as one examination from the University of Copenhagen has demonstrated that expanded supplementation of the cancer prevention agent neutralized the great impacts of activity.

Actually, you don't need to, particularly not to begin. In this day and age we are adapted to be snappy and proficient, and to be brisk we have been acquainted with inexpensive food and handled nourishment.

I think what many individuals foul up as do I (during the time spent fixing my diet) is to think about the nourishment being removed, so obviously with that sort of reasoning it turns out to be almost difficult to go for a super food/rawfood diet. Be that as it may, if we have a go at including the super food/rawfood into our current diet, things like crude vegetables, sprouts, natural products, and juices, you won't experience considerable difficulties exchanging. In the wake of adding these natural products to your diet you may not be as eager and when you're not ravenous, you won't surrender to purchasing inexpensive food and prepared nourishment.

Since you will have more opportunity to consider your buys and you have gotten increasingly acclimated with eating more advantageous. If you need that steak or even a McDonald's cheeseburger, you can get yourself it, and it will taste so much better... or on the other hand you might be fortunate to the point that you won't need it by any stretch of the imagination. When you begin eating Super foods however, you will begin to see how great you feel and the amount more vitality you have, that cheeseburger just won't look as great to you any longer.

During the time spent changing your diet and after change you would like no doubt however, that you're getting enough of the correct sorts of sustenance. Eating Super foods/crude nourishments isn't simply enough you have to do some exploration on the most proficient method to add your fundamental proteins to your new diet. Recall before you got your protein through your meat yet now you need to get it through your vegetables and crude nourishment so you have to recognize what to eat and what blends you have to eat to get enough proteins.

One approach to do this is to present another vegetable or crude dish each week. You have to purchase another vegetable every week and become acclimated to the taste by utilizing it in your feast the entire week. By doing this you will adjust to the new tastes and surfaces and you will begin feeling more regrettable and more terrible for each time you go for inexpensive food or handled nourishment.

CPSIA information can be obtained
at www.ICGtesting.com
Printed in the USA
LVHW040632261020
669801LV00006B/647